LAW AND ETHICS IN BIOMEDICAL RESEARCH: REGULATION, CONFLICT OF INTEREST, AND LIABILITY

Edited by Trudo Lemmens and Duff R. Waring

When a young man named Jesse Gelsinger died in 1999 as a result of his participation in a gene transfer research study, regulatory agencies in the United States began to take a closer look at what was happening in medical research. The publicity surrounding the case and the resulting temporary shutdown of some of the nation's most prestigious academic research centres confirmed what various recent reports in the United States as well as Canada had claimed: that the current systems of regulatory oversight were deeply flawed.

Law and Ethics in Biomedical Research uses the Gelsinger case as a touchstone, illustrating how three major aspects of that case – the flaws in the regulatory system, conflicts of interest, and legal liability – embody the major challenges in the current medical research environment. Editors Trudo Lemmens and Duff R. Waring have brought together top scholars in the field to examine existing models of research review and human subject protection. They demonstrate why these systems are in need of improvement, and explore how legal and regulatory means can be used to strengthen the protection of research subject and safeguard the integrity of research. The volume also addresses the issue of conflict of interest, paying particular attention to the growing commercialization of medical research, as well as the legal liability of scientific investigators, research institutions, and governmental agencies. Liability is a growing concern in medical research and this study is one of the first to explore the legal responsibilities of various parties involved in the research enterprise.

TRUDO LEMMENS is an associate professor in the Faculty of Law at the University of Toronto.

DUFF R. WARING is an assistant professor in the Department of Philosophy at York University.

Edited by
TRUDO LEMMENS AND DUFF R. WARING

Law and Ethics in Biomedical Research: Regulation, Conflict of Interest, and Liability

UNIVERSITY OF TORONTO PRESS
Toronto Buffalo London

University of Toronto Press Incorporated 2006
Toronto Buffalo London
Printed in Canada

ISBN-13: 978-0-8020-8976-2 (cloth)
ISBN-10: 0-8020-8976-3 (cloth)

ISBN-13: 978-0-8020-8643-3 (paper)
ISBN-10: 0-8020-8643-8 (paper)

∞

Printed on acid-free paper

Library and Archives Canada Cataloguing in Publication

Law and ethics in biomedical research : regulation, conflict of interest
and liability / edited by Trudo Lemmens and Duff Waring.

Includes bibliographical references and index
ISBN-13: 978-0-8020-8976-2 (bound)
ISBN-10: 0-8020-8976-3 (bound)
ISBN-13: 978-0-8020-8643-2 (pbk.)
ISBN-10: 0-8020-8643-8 (pbk.)

1. Medicine – Research – Law and legislation – United States.   2. Medicine –
Research – Law and legislation – Canada.   3. Human experimentation in
medicine – United States.   4. Human experimentation in medicine –
Canada.   5. Medicine – Research – Moral and ethical aspects –
United States.   6. Medicine – Research – Moral and ethical aspects –
Canada.   I. Lemmens, Trudo   II. Waring, Duff William Ramus, 1955–

KE3663.M38L39 2006   344.7304'196   C2005-905941-9
KF3827.M38L39 2006

University of Toronto Press acknowledges the financial assistance to
its publishing program of the Canada Council for the Arts and the
Ontario Arts Council.

University of Toronto Press acknowledges the financial support for its
publishing activities of the Government of Canada through the Book
Publishing Industry Development Program (BPIDP).

This book is respectfully dedicated to the memory of
Jesse Gelsinger

Contents

Acknowledgments

The editors gratefully acknowledge Genome Canada through the Ontario Genomics Institute for its generous support throughout the production of this volume, and for sponsoring the conference held in November 2002 from which the idea for this book and many of the chapters in it originated.

We thank *Guinea Pig Zero*, the Hastings Center, and the *Journal of Law, Medicine and Ethics* for their kind permission to include revised versions of articles that now constitute chapters 1, 3, and 7 of this collection.

We are grateful to Angela Long, Agape Lim, and Tony Cheung for their dedicated research assistance, to Tom Archibald for helping to prepare the index, and to Linda Hutjens for copy-editing and management of the project.

We would like to thank Stephen Kotowych and Virgil Duff of the University of Toronto Press for their encouragement and guidance at various stages in the process.

Trudo Lemmens thanks his wife, Pascale Chapdelaine, and his sons, Rafaël and Albéric, for their love, and for their understanding when work sometimes interfered with family life.

Duff Waring thanks his wife, Jayne Davis, and his brother, Michael Waring, for their ongoing support.

LAW AND ETHICS IN BIOMEDICAL RESEARCH

Introduction

TRUDO LEMMENS AND DUFF R. WARING

Research ethics has developed in the shadow of controversy. Throughout the twentieth century, various scandals prompted professional organizations, governmental agencies, and courts to look closely at how medical research was being conducted and how the well-being of human research subjects could be better protected. The Nuremberg Doctors' Trial and names such as Tuskegee, Willowbrook, and the Brooklyn Jewish Chronic Disease Hospital have become enshrined in the collective consciousness of the medical research community as dire symbols of how, in their zeal to conduct research, physician investigators can ignore the welfare of patients. These scandals concerned studies involving vulnerable persons at the margins of society, such as prisoners, people with disabilities, children, or patients at the end of life, several of whom were exposed to serious physical suffering or significant risk of harm. Participants in these controversial studies seldom gave meaningful consent.

The public outcry and professional debates that followed the exposure of such scandals pushed the research community to develop reforms. International and national ethics guidelines were promulgated and procedures to scrutinize studies with human subjects were put in place. As a result, review by independent review boards – referred to as Institutional Review Boards (IRBs) in the United States, and Research Ethics Boards (REBs) in Canada – became firmly entrenched as a necessary precondition for human subjects research. These review boards received the professional mandate to protect the rights and well-being of research subjects. Among other things, they evaluate the scientific validity and value of proposed research, weigh its risks and potential benefits and determine whether informed consent procedures are appropriate.

In the last two decades, however, various reports have stressed that the current system of research oversight, with its reliance on lightly regulated and largely volunteer boards, is in need of improvement. In 1995, a voluminous report by the U.S. President's Advisory Committee on Human Radiation Experiments revealed that the research review system did not prevent ethically troubling projects from being promoted by the government and then approved by various REBs. It recommended several changes to this system. Other recent reports by the U.S. Office of the Inspector General and by the National Bioethics Advisory Commission have also claimed that the research review system is in jeopardy. In Canada, three federal funding agencies took the initiative to improve the basis for research ethics review in 1998 by introducing a new *Tri-Council Policy Statement on Research Involving Humans.* Despite this and other initiatives aimed at raising the standards of ethical scrutiny, various commentators and a 2001 Law Commission of Canada report have emphasized flaws in the Canadian system of research review that are at least as serious as those in the United States.

Research controversies still send the clearest signal that human subjects may not be sufficiently protected and that additional safeguards are needed. Among recent controversies, the Jesse Gelsinger case stands out. The tragic story of this young man is a connecting thread of this collection, which explores the potential role of law in advancing both the protection of human research subjects and the integrity of science.

The Gelsinger case is paradigmatic for at least three reasons. First, it occurred notwithstanding the oversight of an experienced IRB, thus exposing serious limitations of the current review system. Second, the investigators and the institution in which the research took place had significant commercial interests in the study's outcome. These interests appear to have influenced how the study was promoted and how the investigators behaved once Jesse was enrolled as a subject. Finally, the Gelsinger case led to liability claims against the investigators and their institution. Although the case was settled out of court, the claims made in this case illustrate the possibility of legal action against researchers and against individual scientists and research institutions.

Paul Gelsinger once trusted the research establishment and shared with his son Jesse the view that volunteering as a research subject was a personal contribution to the life-saving potential of medicine. The book commences with Paul Gelsinger's personal account of what he and his family endured when Jesse died in a highly controversial gene therapy trial. One of the striking outcomes of this story is the way in which it transformed a proud father into a staunch critic of commercialized research and a strong advocate for stricter regulation. Paul Gelsinger's narrative powerfully depicts major flaws in the regulation of medical research and puts all-too-human faces on a topic that might otherwise be dismissed as academic. All those who have heard Paul Gelsinger tell this story in person will attest that it is a moving experience. His testimony exemplifies and personalizes the fundamental reasons why we ought to pay more attention to regulation, conflict of interest, and liability in biomedical research.

These topics are characteristic of the new research environment and provide the three-part structure of this book. In the first part, U.S. and Canadian scholars describe the status of research regulation and oversight in these two countries. They emphasize the changes that have taken place in the regulation of medical research and the contexts in which calls for improvement are now occurring. The second part of the book addresses conflicts of interest, with particular attention to the growing commercialization of medical research. Chapter 7 explores legal and regulatory means to deal with certain commercial research practices. Legal remedies are the focus of the third part of this book. The legal liability of scientific investigators, research institutions, and governmental agencies is the focus of analysis. Legal liability is a growing concern in medical research and we are among the first to explore the liability of various parties involved in the research enterprise.

The chapters on regulation begin with Kathleen Cranley Glass's picture of the Canadian system of research governance as fragmented, decentralized, and lacking an accountable system of ethics review. REBs currently operate without a systemic infrastructure for the education of members, the monitoring of board reviews, or the accreditation of their functions. She notes fourteen research governance issues that should be addressed by a national system for the governance of research involving humans, including the fact that 'increased demands for review are being placed on REBs without making corresponding resources available.' These are practical issues that will require significant investments of human, administrative, and financial resources. They also require the political commitment to create a system of research governance that is truly independent of the private sector's growing financial interests in the biomedical technology industry. That commitment seems to be gathering as much dust as the federal government's pledge in the 2002 Throne Speech to 'work with the provinces to implement a national system for the governance of research involving humans, including national research ethics and standards.' As Professor Glass notes in her conclusion, there have been no government proposals for the establishment of such a national system, even though more fragmented initiatives have been undertaken by various agencies involved in the protection of human subjects.

A U.S. perspective is provided by Anna Mastroianni and Jeffrey Kahn, both of whom were major contributors to the aforementioned President's Advisory Committee on Human Radiation Experiments. The authors trace the shifting application of justice in U.S. federal policies on biomedical research with human subjects. The regulatory 'culture' that stressed protection from risk in the 1970s began to shift in the late 1980s to stress access to, and fair distribution of, the prospective benefits of research. Advocacy groups, especially those representing women with breast cancer and people with AIDS, argued that the cutting edge of therapy was in research participation. The notion of justice as protection thus shifted to the notion of justice as access. The authors conclude that the pendulum may have swung as far as it can towards the emphasis on benefits and is now swinging back towards protection. They suggest that we now confront a culture of institutional caution and an 'overemphasis' on regulatory compliance. They indicate an emerging approach to research that emphasizes partnership between those who conduct research, those who oversee it, and those who participate as subjects. This approach revolves around a culture devoted to the maintenance of trust between these parties. Such an approach might balance the pendulum's swing between protection and access by supporting both appropriate protections and fair access to benefits.

It should come as no surprise that we devote four chapters in the second part of the book to conflict of interest. The potential impact of this topic on the public's trust in science, as well as the fact that two of the more notorious disputes around conflicts of interest have shaken up the academic institution in which we work, have motivated our concern. The controversies surrounding Dr Nancy Olivieri's research findings and her struggle with the pharmaceutical company Apotex, as well as the denial of employment to Dr David Healy, a noted critic of industry-sponsored research into psychiatric drugs, only increase the need for critical reflection on this topic at the University of Toronto.

The controversies in Toronto have spurred important debates, not only in the Canadian academic community, but outside North America. They are invoked in these chapters as examples of the real or perceived impact of the commercialization of medical research on academic freedom and scientific integrity. The conference on which this book is based and the various contributions to it are a reflection of the possibility of critical and constructive debate on these highly charged issues, a debate which is a fundamental part of academic life.

The first chapter in this section begins with Sheldon Krimsky's analysis of the ethical and legal foundations of conflict of interest in the sciences. He notes that 'conflict of interest' is a relatively new term to the scientific and medical research communities, having attracted little attention before the 1980s. Lawyers understand well that conflict of interest can be an ethical problem in various legal procedures; it can, for instance, erode the goal of a fair trial. But in what sense is conflict of interest an ethical problem among scientists? Krimsky argues that it can erode scientific integrity, which involves organized scepticism, objectivity, disinterestedness, and a willingness to disagree openly about conflicting results. All of these elements can be compromised as science is commercialized in the private interest. Moreover, the ethical and legal measures needed to protect scientific integrity require more than mere disclosure of conflicting interests; they require measures that clearly separate roles. For example, the roles of academic researchers should be separate and distinct from the roles of those who have a financial interest in the knowledge they produce. From our perspective, what Krimsky calls 'science in the private interest' should be offset by national standards of review that serve the public interest in safe, trustworthy research.

James Robert Brown examines an issue seldom explored in the literature on conflict of interest: the self-censorship that researchers and institutions may impose on themselves to safeguard their commercial interests in the knowledge they produce. For this reason, some types of research will not be pursued, or, if pursued, will not be reported. Brown regards this problem as beyond the reach of regulation or law. Regulation might ensure that any research that is published meets a threshold of scientific legitimacy. It might, that is, prove effective in the prevention of fraudulent reporting. But Brown claims that there is nothing that any journal or regulatory body can do about self-censorship. His proposal for reform – a return to public funding for all medical research – seems radical. But it may tell us much about the current context of medical research that such a proposal can be considered radical.

Lorraine Ferris and David Naylor describe a number of threats to the integrity of industry-sponsored clinical trials that arise from conflict of interest. Evidence of the pharmaceutical industry's influence on the design, conduct, analysis, and reporting of new drug trials inspires growing concern about the validity of evidence used for assessing their safety and efficacy. The authors review some of the remedies implemented in Canada but note that we have fallen behind the United States in terms of legislation and regulation to deal systematically with conflict of interest issues. They offer a number of recommendations to manage conflict of interest in industry-sponsored trials. These include the creation of consistent policies for all Canadian academic health science centres, the mandatory declaration of conflict of interest by investigators and research sites to Health Canada's Therapeutic Products Directorate before research is allowed to proceed, a governance model for REBs that is entrenched in federal legislation, and an adequate national inspection strategy for clinical trials.

Trudo Lemmens and Paul B. Miller deal with a subject that exemplifies the increasingly competitive nature of medical research: the use of financial recruitment incentives, a practice especially prevalent in clinical drug trials. While it has received some attention in the medical literature, few authors have situated this practice within the larger context of commercialized research. Fewer still have described the legal recourses available to deal with it. As the authors indicate, the rapid recruitment of subjects has become one of the most significant challenges to an expanding research industry. Direct and indirect financial recruitment incentives have an impact on both scientific integrity and the protection of research subjects. They can also influence the overall direction of research. This phenomenon calls for a regulatory response. While acknowledging that ethics guidelines and professional codes of ethics – which generally frown upon the practice – may have some persuasive moral force, Lemmens and Miller argue that there is currently too much reliance on the work of largely unregulated research ethics boards. They suggest that more stringent legal means can be employed, including the use of professional regulations related to conflicts of interest, the common law doctrine of fiduciary duty, and even criminal law provisions related to fraud. The chapter concludes with a call for a fundamental change in the regulatory structure surrounding drug or medical device research, the area of research in which financial recruitment incentives are most prevalent. Lemmens and Miller discuss how the proposal to establish an independent national drug agency that would itself coordinate and directly control clinical trials would also curb the problems related to the use of financial recruitment incentives. The negative impact of commercial interests on research requires us to think about a strict separation between those who have financial interests in the outcome of research and those who conduct the research. This recommendation deserves attention, especially in light of the recent controversies surrounding the efficacy and safety of a variety of drugs.

While potential liability is already evoked in the last chapter of the second part of the book, the third section focuses specifically on legal liability. Little has been written about the potential legal liability of research scientists, the institutions at which their studies are conducted, or the REBs or IRBs which review them. The section on liability offers some preliminary explorations of this controversial area. Mary Thomson examines the liability of those pursuing gene transfer (or 'gene therapy') research with human subjects. Since the death of Jesse Gelsinger, researchers and their sponsors have effectively been put on notice that they risk being named in lawsuits if human subjects are harmed as a result of their participation in gene transfer trials. Thomson's discussion of the deaths of Jesse Gelsinger and James Dent provides a useful framework in which to examine the potential for liability. How might a court assess situations involving death or harm to trial participants, especially if informed consent has been shown to be compromised? In her view, the sponsors, researchers, research institutions, and review boards will hold the balance of knowledge about adverse events and the various financial interests that might be involved in a trial. Given the higher legal standard of informed consent in research, indications of conflict of interest, and the fiduciary duty owed to research participants, Thomson argues that courts will most likely expect defendants to refute responsibility for such tragic outcomes.

Waring and Glass examine the potential liability of researchers for harm to research subjects in the placebo arm of a drug trial. How could a court decide such a case with relevant legal principles and available case law? The authors begin their analysis by evaluating the administration of placebos with regard to existing malpractice law. A key argument here is their claim that the therapeutic obligations of physicians providing treatment should apply to medical researchers. According to

Waring and Glass, administering placebos to patients who become research participants can amount to practising substandard medicine. They also argue that the enrolment of ill persons who seek established, effective treatment might constitute a separate claim for breach of fiduciary duty. The research participant's voluntary assumption of risk through informed consent may not justify such a breach, but the main thrust of the authors' analysis is not the failure to adequately inform. Rather, it is the failure to offer research participants treatment when there is an effective therapy for their condition.

Finally, Sana Halwani considers the potential liability of the Crown for research activities funded or regulated by the federal government. While her analysis of negligence is based on general tort and Crown liability principles, her chapter is focused practically on claims that could be made against two federal funding agencies: the Canadian Institutes of Health Research and the Therapeutic Products Directorate. She notes numerous obstacles in bringing a lawsuit against the Crown for injury resulting from research that it has funded or authorized. Major hurdles to plaintiffs include establishing a 'novel duty' from research reviewer to research subject and showing that the act or omission was not part of a Crown policy that limits the scope of potential liability. While a research subject could argue that such a policy is unreasonable, courts are not usually receptive to such arguments, especially if the policy can be justified by underlying economic and political reasons.

Although this collection is part of the larger literature related to biomedical research ethics, we wanted analyses of legal and regulatory issues to predominate. There are currently few books dealing exclusively with the legal aspects of research regulation, and we have attempted to fill part of that void. We also intend our legal focus to send a message. As noted above, the Jesse Gelsinger case accentuates the need for a more stringent regulatory system in a world of increasingly commercialized, for-profit research. New directions in biomedical research deal with many unknown variables and may involve invasive procedures on seriously ill patients. Gene transfer and forthcoming clinical trials involving stem cells are two prominent examples. It can be expected that more serious adverse events will be associated with some of this research. Some level of risk may be unavoidable, but it is crucial that what happened to Jesse Gelsinger does not happen again.

While the uncertainty inherent in much new biomedical research makes it hard to avoid all potential mishaps, a firmer review structure, coupled with stricter regulation of conflicts of interest, might go a long way towards enhancing the protection of research subjects. This approach might also help to preserve public trust in research science. As some of the contributors to this book indicate, potential tort liability for research misconduct also lurks in the background when professional standards are not respected. It is our hope that this collection will contribute to further debate and inspire those who question the rationale behind research regulation. We believe that various chapters demonstrate convincingly that research regulation not only aims at protecting the rights and well-being of human subjects but also to protect the ethical foundations of science and the institutions in which scientific research is practised.

While medical research has been integrated into a competitive commercial environment, it is still too often approached as if it were purely driven by humanistic ideals. We hope that the discussion in this book will contribute to the establishment of a more coherent and firm regulatory and legal structure to shape this important societal endeavour.

1 Uninformed Consent: The Case of Jesse Gelsinger

PAUL L. GELSINGER

It has been four years since we first became involved with a clinical research protocol for gene therapy conducted at the University of Pennsylvania (Penn). Penn, the oldest medical university in the United States, had established the Institute for Human Gene Therapy (IHGT) in 1992. In the spring of 1993 James Wilson, MD, PhD, was lured to Penn to head the IHGT. It was hoped that Dr Wilson's endeavours there would open the doors into a new and promising field of medicine. The premise and the promise of gene therapy would bring untold fame and wealth to those able to make it a reality.

Under my guidance, my son, Jesse Gelsinger, participated in one of the gene transfer clinical trials being conducted at Dr Wilson's institute. In June of 2000, I wrote a piece titled 'Jesse's Intent'[1] at the request of Bob Helms, editor of *Guinea Pig Zero*, a small journal published in an effort to expose the problems of clinical research. Jesse's story is real and should help all of us realize what is most important in our lives.

Jesse's Intent

Born on 18 June 1981, Jesse Gelsinger was a real character in a lot of ways. Not having picked out a name for him prior to his birth, the name Jesse came to us three days later. When considering a middle name, we pondered James but decided that just 'Jesse' was enough for this kid. His infancy was pretty normal. With a brother thirteen months his senior, he was not overly spoiled. He crawled and walked at the appropriate ages. When he started talking, it quickly became obvious that this was one kid who would speak his mind and crack everybody up at the same time. He nursed until he was nearly two years old.

It wasn't until Jesse was about two years and eight months old that his metabolic disorder reared its ugly head. Jesse had always been a very picky eater. Since weaning, he increasingly refused to eat meat and dairy products, focusing instead on potatoes and cereals. After the birth of his sister in late January 1984 and following a mild cold in March, Jesse's behaviour became very erratic over a brief period of time. Because his mother had previously experienced schizophrenic symptoms, I was concerned that Jesse might be exhibiting signs of psychosis. His speech was very belligerent, as if possessed. My wife, Pattie, and I took him to see our family doctor. Thinking that Jesse was anaemic because of his poor diet and lethargy, he put Jesse on a high-protein diet. It turns out that that was the worst thing for Jesse. Forcing him to eat peanut butter sandwiches and bacon and to drink milk over the next two days overwhelmed Jesse's system.

On a Saturday in mid-March 1984 Jesse awoke, parked himself in front of the television to watch cartoons, and promptly fell back asleep. When we were unable to rouse him, we became alarmed. His mother called the doctor and insisted that we be allowed to take Jesse to Children's Hospital of Philadelphia (CHOP), just across the Delaware River from our home near Woodbury, New Jersey. Upon arrival at CHOP, Jesse was admitted through the emergency room in what they called a first stage coma. He responded to stimuli but would not awaken. After several tests indicated high blood ammonia, the doctor told us that Jesse most probably had Reye's syndrome, which upset us very much. Several hours later they indicated that other tests indicated that this was not Reye's and that they would need to run more tests to determine what was wrong with Jesse. Within a week, we had the diagnosis of ornithine transcarbamylase deficiency syndrome (OTC). We were told that OTC is a very rare metabolic disorder. Jesse's form of the disorder was considered mild and could be controlled by medication and diet.

And so, after eleven days in the hospital, Jesse came home and we watched like hawks everything he ate and made certain that he took his medications. From there on Jesse progressed fairly normally, although he was small for his age. It wasn't until he was ten that he would need to be hospitalized again for his disorder. Following a weekend of too much protein intake, Jesse's system was unable to rid itself of the ammonia build-up fast enough and he again slipped into a coma. His specialist scrambled to find a way to make him well again, never having had to treat hyperammonemia before. But within five days, Jesse was well enough to go home, having suffered no apparent neurological damage.

As Jesse entered his teenage years he resisted taking his medications. He felt that he could control his disorder and only took his medications when he didn't feel well. His mother and I divorced in 1989, two years after our move to Tucson, Arizona, and Jesse was under my care after I obtained custody of my four children in 1990. At age sixteen, he was taking nearly fifty pills a day to control his illness. I remarried in 1992. My new wife, Mickie, and I kept a careful watch on Jesse, but as he grew older, we expected him to take more care of himself. With six children between us, we had many demands on our time. Jesse was being seen at a state-funded metabolic clinic in Tucson twice a year to monitor his development and, while not always compliant, he was progressing into adulthood.

In September 1998, Jesse and I were made aware by his specialist of a clinical trial being done at the University of Pennsylvania in Philadelphia. People were working on what the specialist described as 'gene therapy' for Jesse's disorder. We were instantly interested, but Jesse was told that he could not participate until age eighteen. That same fall, Jesse was stressing his metabolism as he had never done before, having recently acquired a part-time job and an off-road motorcycle. I saw little of him. As a senior in high school, Jesse had a very busy schedule. Unknown to me at the time, he was experiencing symptoms of his disorder but trying to hide them. He didn't want any restrictions placed on his activities. I knew that he was inconsistent in taking his medications because I rarely had to order them, and I spoke with him every other week about his need to take better care of himself. It took nearly dying to convince him of this.

On 22 December 1998, I arrived home in mid-afternoon to find Jesse curled up on the couch. A close friend was with him. Jesse was very frightened. He was vomiting uncontrollably and could not hold down his medications. After about five minutes with him, I determined that I could not manage his recovery. I convinced his paediatrician and specialist that Jesse needed to be hospitalized and placed on intravenous fluids. With his ammonia levels at six times the normal level, Jesse was in trouble. After no significant changes in his condition by 24 December, the hospital let Jesse go home for Christmas. Listless all day, Jesse crashed Christmas night and was admitted to intensive care where they discovered hypoglycemia, seriously low blood sugar. His specialist felt certain that it was due to one of his medications, l-arginine, and discontinued it. He also decided that Jesse's primary medication, sodium benzoate, was not effective enough and ordered that a newer, better medication be provided.

Jesse recovered well enough to be placed in a regular room at the hospital, but his ammonia levels refused to drop. I was staying in the hospital at Jesse's side day and night. Two days after Christmas, on a Sunday afternoon, Jesse and I had a conversation about how he was doing. I described to Jesse how it seemed that he was stuck up a tree, not knowing whether he was going to climb down or fall out. I went home to be with the rest of my family and sleep in my own bed for a night. Jesse called me at about 11 P.M. and said, 'Dad, I fell out of the tree.' He was again vomiting uncontrollably. I rushed back to the hospital and spent a heart-rending two days trying to help my son through his crisis. On Monday, I discovered that the insurance company was baulking at paying for Jesse's new medications and that they had not been shipped. I told the pharmacist to purchase the new medications ($3,300 for one month's supply) with my credit card and that I would deal with the insurance company later. At that point, the insurance company relented and authorized the medications; they were ordered on Tuesday. By Tuesday afternoon, 29 December, Jesse was so listless that I grew very alarmed that he would not get well.

At 5 p.m., Jesse began to vomit again and he was becoming incoherent. I moved into the hall to get help; there I found his paediatrician examining his chart. I summoned him to Jesse's room and while he called in the intensive care doctor, I called my wife and told her to come immediately. Jesse's aunt and grandmother arrived for a visit only to find Jesse in a crisis. Mickie arrived and together we held Jesse while they prepared a bed for him in intensive care. The intensive care doctor, seeing Jesse's deteriorating condition and believing him to be mentally impaired, inquired if life support would be appropriate. I realized that these people had not known Jesse well, and explained that the loss of mental faculties that they were seeing was not Jesse's normal state at all. Jesse developed tremors and began to vomit, then, suddenly he just stopped. I whispered to Mickie, 'He's still breathing, isn't he?' I asked Jesse's paediatrician to check him. After placing his stethoscope on Jesse's chest for a few moments he looked to the nurse present and told her to call a code blue. We were whisked from the room, while they intubated and manually ventilated our son and took him to intensive care. We were distraught, believing Jesse to be near death. After fifteen minutes they indicated that they were getting him under control, that his heart had never stopped.

For two days, Jesse lingered in an induced coma to allow the ventilator to control his breathing. He weighed in at only ninety-seven pounds, down from his healthy weight of 120 pounds. His old medication only partially lowered his ammonia level. On Thursday morning Jesse's new medications arrived. They were administered through a gastrointestinal feed, and within twenty-four hours, Jesse's ammonia levels started falling. We waited at his side as he began to regain consciousness. His first conscious act was to motion us to change the television station. Jesse was back! Within a day he was out of intensive care, with normal ammonia levels, something he had never known his entire life. He was ordering and eating food like a teenager, something else he had never experienced. We were ecstatic. When his specialist came to see him, I shook his hand and told him that he had a medical miracle on his hands. A week after nearly dying, Jesse was back in school full-time with a newfound zeal for life.

By early February 1999 Jesse had recovered enough strength to consider returning to work, but he came down with a serious case of influenza. Because illness often triggered Jesse's metabolic disorder, I stayed home to keep an eye on his condition. Jesse was kind enough to pass the bug on to me. It was the sickest I'd been in twenty years, with fever for six days and fatigue for four weeks. Jesse recovered within a week and was back in school. I had him tested twice while he was ill and his ammonia level was only slightly elevated. The new meds were working wonderfully.

Near the end of February, Jesse returned to his part-time job as a courtesy clerk at a supermarket three miles from our home. On Saturday the twenty-seventh, he called me at 11 p.m. for a ride home. I picked him up in my work van and, on the way home, we had a fateful conversation. I had been asking Jesse to find out if his job would offer him medical insurance once he graduated from school in May. Being a typical teenager, he had done nothing to inquire and I told him in no uncertain terms that he needed medical insurance if he wasn't going to continue his education. At the time, we believed that Jesse would not be covered under our insurance once he left school.

Jesse rarely raged at his illness but this time he flung a half-full bottle of soda against my windshield while cursing his disorder. In anger, I gave him a backhand punch to the shoulder and chastised him. Only two blocks from home, Jesse in anger flung open the door and told me he was jumping out. I said, 'Whoa, wait until I stop.' As I was coming to a stop he gave me a look like he was jumping and went out the door. All I could envision was Jesse falling under the van and me running him over. Sure enough, even though I had nearly stopped, he fell. As I stopped, I could hear him screaming that I was on his arm. Now, my work van is loaded with tools and weighs six thousand pounds. Thinking, 'Oh God, No!' I threw the van in park and raced around the back to find Jesse's right arm and elbow pinned under the right rear tire. Making certain that his body was clear, I rolled the van forward off his arm. The kid was crying in agony. As I cradled him in my arms, I cried, 'You idiot, what were you thinking' and then 'Jesse, I'm sorry.' With Jesse begging me not to move him, I knew he would need an ambulance. His arm was a red mess from wrist to upper arm with the elbow area gouged out. The tire print was evident on the underside of his arm.

As I began to think about seeking help, a woman who had witnessed what happened while driving from the other direction asked if she could help. I told her to please call 911 and she drove off to do so. A neighbour, hearing the commotion, came out and offered his help. Another passerby offered me his cell phone and I called my wife. Within minutes, the paramedics arrived, strapped Jesse to a gurney, and whisked him off to the hospital. After the police informed me that I had done no wrong, that I could not control his actions, it was all I could do to drive the one block left to get home. I had helped Jesse through his near-death experience in December and through a serious bout with the flu only to nearly end his life in an accident.

Shaking and emotional, my wife Mickie drove me to the hospital. Jesse was okay; he hadn't even broken his arm! While suffering extensive road rash and a serious wound to his elbow he recovered full use of his arm following two days in the hospital and a month of physical therapy. I was an emotional wreck for a week following the accident. This kid was something else. His sister told him that if he caused me to have a heart attack she was going to kill him. A month later I got word from our insurance company regarding Jesse's status if he did not continue his education. He was covered until age twenty-five as long as he remained our dependant. I joked with him that I had run him over for nothing. He was proud of his war wound with dad. God, what a relief it was to see this kid bounce back again.

In early April 1999, Jesse again had an appointment at the metabolic clinic. While there, the subject of gene therapy and the clinical trial at the University of Pennsylvania came up again. Jesse and I were both still very interested. I informed the doctor that we were already planning a trip to New Jersey in late June, that Jesse would be eighteen at that time, and to let Penn know that we were interested. I received a letter from Penn in April, firming things up and by late May, our visit was set. We would fly in on 18 June and Jesse would be tested on the twenty-second. Jesse was none too happy about flying in on the eighteenth; that was his birthday and he wanted to party with his friends. But a few days later he told me it was okay. I said that it was a good thing since I had already bought the tickets for all six of us a month earlier.

So, on Friday, 18 June 1999, Jesse, his three siblings, PJ (age nineteen), Mary (fifteen), and Anne (fourteen), and Mickie and I boarded a plane to take us down a path we never imagined. We had a party for Jesse that night at my brother's house and a reunion with ten of my fifteen siblings and extended families that Sunday. It was great to see everyone. The kids got to meet cousins they hadn't seen in twelve years. Jesse's cousins nicknamed him Captain Kirk for the way he struck the volleyball with a two-handed chop. This was turning into a great vacation.

We hung out on Monday and on Tuesday, 22 June, we all headed over to Philly to meet with the clinical trial people. We arrived a few minutes late because of a wrong turn on the expressway, only to discover that they weren't ready for us. The nurse in charge rounded up Dr Raper and after a forty-five-minute wait we were ushered into a hospital room to go over consent forms and discuss the procedures that Jesse would undergo. Dr Raper described the technique that would be used: Jesse would be sedated and two catheters would be placed into his liver; one in the hepatic artery at the inlet to the liver to inject the viral vector and another to monitor the blood exiting the liver to ensure that the vector was all being absorbed by the liver. He explained the dangers associated with this and that Jesse would need to remain immobile for about eight hours after the infusion to minimize the risk of a clot breaking free from the infusion site.

Dr Raper also explained that Jesse would experience flu-like symptoms for a few days. He briefly explained that there was a remote possibility of contracting hepatitis. When I questioned him on this, he explained that hepatitis was just an inflammation of the liver and that the liver was a remarkable organ, the only organ in the body with the ability to regenerate itself. In reading the consent form, I noticed the

possibility of a liver transplant being required if the hepatitis progressed. The hepatitis seemed such a rare possibility and the need for
transplant even more remote that no more alarms went off in my head.
Dr Raper proceeded to the next phase and what appeared the most
dangerous aspect of the testing. A needle biopsy of Jesse's liver was to
be performed one week after the infusion. Numbers explaining the
risks of uncontrolled side effects were included. There was a one in ten
thousand chance that Jesse could die of the biopsy. I told Jesse that he
needed to read and understand what he was getting into, that this was
serious stuff. The risks seemed very remote but also very real. Still, one
in ten thousand weren't bad odds in my mind. There would be no benefit to Jesse, Dr Raper explained. Even if the genes worked, the effect
would be transient: the body's immune system would attack and kill
the virus over a four- to six-week period.

After our forty-five-minute conversation with Dr Raper ended, Jesse
consented to undergo the five-hour N15 ammonia study to determine
his level of enzyme efficiency. Many vials of blood were taken before
Jesse drank a small vial of N15 ammonia. This special isotope of
ammonia would then show up in Jesse's blood and urine. The rate at
which it was processed out of the body would determine Jesse's efficiency. Going into this study we were aware that Jesse's efficiency was
only 6 per cent of that of a normal person.

After waiting with Jesse for two hours the family decided to head
out to Pat's Steaks for lunch and tour South Street for a few hours. On
our return to the hospital, Jesse was finished and ready to leave. It was
now mid-afternoon and we decided to see the Betsy Ross house and
Independence Mall. After checking out the Liberty Bell, the kids
wanted to see the Rocky statue, so we headed over to the Art Museum.
Four of us, Jesse, PJ, Mary, and me, raced up the steps Rocky-style (we
had watched the movie the night before). Finding only Rocky's foot-
steps, we learned that the statue had been moved to the Spectrum and
headed over to Pattison Avenue. A Phillies game was about to start, so
I stayed in our rented Durango while the kids had their pictures taken
by Mickie. It was a fun time for everyone, especially Jesse. He was
starting to feel good about what he was doing. This was his thing and
he had a chance to help. The following day, we toured New York City.
Everybody got to pick a place to visit. Jesse chose FAO Schwartz toy,
store where he bought four pro-wrestling action figures. We all had a
great day, finishing with the Empire State Building and the Staten
Island Ferry.

Four weeks later, back in Tucson, we received a letter addressed to Mr Paul Gelsinger and Jesse. It was from Dr Mark Batshaw confirming Jesse's 6 per cent efficiency of OTC and stating that they would like to have Jesse in their study. I presented the letter to Jesse and asked him if he still wanted to do this. He hesitated a moment, and said yes. Dr Batshaw called about a week later to follow up on his letter and spoke to Jesse briefly. Jesse told him that he would need to talk everything over with me and call back. Jesse was deferring to my understanding and Dr Batshaw was well aware of that.

When I spoke to Dr Batshaw, we discussed a number of things. Since they had forgotten to include the graph showing Jesse's N15 results, he faxed it to us. I asked if Jesse was the least efficient patient in the study. Dr Batshaw confirmed that he was. Dr Batshaw steered the conversation to the results they had experienced to date. He explained that they had shown that the treatment had worked temporarily in mice, even preventing death in mice exposed to lethal injections of ammonia. He then explained that the most recent patient had shown a 50 per cent increase in her ability to excrete ammonia following gene therapy. My reaction was to say, 'Wow Mark! This really works. So, with Jesse at 6 per cent efficiency you may be able to show exactly how well this works.' His response was that that was their hope and that it would be for these kids. He explained that another twenty-five liver disorders could be treated with the same technique, and that overall these disorders affected about one in every five hundred people. I did some quick math and figured that's 500,000 people in the United States alone, 12,000,000 worldwide. I dropped my guard. Dr Batshaw and I never discussed the dangerous side of this work. When I presented Dr Batshaw's remarks to Jesse, he knew the right thing to do: he signed on to help everybody and, hopefully, himself in the long run. The plan was for him to be the last patient tested and he was tentatively scheduled for mid-October.

By late July 1999 Jesse had a new focus for his life, but he also had other priorities. He had acquired a tattoo on the back of his right calf, without discussing it with me first, and he had used the money he owed me to get it done! I had just bought him a used street motorcycle as a graduation present and he was getting his driver's licence, which he obtained on 21 August. It was wonderful to see him grinning ear to ear as he drove off on his bike for the first time. We saw little of Jesse over the next two weeks. If he wasn't working, he was out riding with his buddy, Gar, or spending the night at a friend's house. He was still living at home and paying thirty-five dollars a week for rent and fifteen dollars a week for the bike insurance we had fronted for him. This kid was really living and we were so proud of him.

In mid-August Penn told us that they were having trouble scheduling their next patient, and asked if Jesse would be available in September. I explained that I would have to check with him. He okayed it and arranged to take an unpaid leave of absence. Most communications with Penn were done via e-mail at this point. The finalized date of admission would be 9 September, 1999. I wanted to go with Jesse, but being self-employed and not seeing any great danger, I scheduled to fly in for what I had perceived as the most dangerous aspect of the testing, the liver biopsy. I would fly in on the eighteenth and return with Jesse on the twenty-first.

As 9 September approached, everyone became more and more focused on Jesse's trip: Mickie bought him some new clothes; Jesse assembled his pro-wrestling, Sylvester Stallone, and Adam Sandler videos; and I worked like a dog to get as much done as possible in preparation for my own departure. With one bag of videos and another with clothing, Jesse and I headed off to the airport early on Thursday the ninth. He was both apprehensive and excited. He had to change planes in Phoenix and hail a cab for the hospital once he arrived in Philly. Jesse had never been away from Tucson on his own prior to this trip. Words cannot express how proud I was of him. Just eighteen, he was going off to help the world. As I walked him to his gate, I gave him a big hug, looked him in the eye, and told him he was my hero. When I drove off to work, I thought of him and what he was doing, and started considering how to get him some recognition. Little did I know what effect this kid was going to have.

Jesse called us that night using his phone card. He was well, but had had a little mix-up with the cabbie about which hospital he was going to. The cabbie was cool about it though, he said. The cabbie reminded him of a scary version of James Earl Jones. Jesse was to have more N15 testing the following day and again on Sunday before the actual gene infusion on Monday, 13 September. Saturday was an off day and he would be able to leave the hospital. Two of my brothers had arranged to visit with Jesse and that had put me at ease about not going. Jesse had a blast with his uncle and cousins on Saturday and a good visit with his other uncle and aunt on Sunday. Mickie and I spoke with Jesse every day and his spirits were good. He was apprehensive on Sunday evening. Dr Raper had put him on intravenous medications because his ammonia was elevated. I reasoned with him that these guys knew what they were doing, that they knew more about OTC than anybody on the planet. I didn't talk with the doctors; it was late.

I received a call from Dr Raper on Monday, just after they infused Jesse. He explained that everything went well and that Jesse would return to his room in a few hours. I discussed the infusion and how the vector did its job. Dr Raper didn't like my use of the word 'invade' when I explained what I thought the virus did to the liver cells. He explained that if they could affect about 1 per cent of Jesse's cells, then they would get the results they desired. Mickie and I spoke with Jesse later that evening. He had the expected fever and was not feeling well. I told him to hang in there, that I loved him. He responded, 'I love you too, dad.' Mickie got the same kind of goodbye. Little did we know it was our last.

I awoke very early Tuesday morning and went to work. I received a mid-morning call from Steve Raper asking if Jesse had a history of jaundice. I told him 'not since he was first born.' He explained that Jesse was jaundiced and a bit disoriented. I said, 'That's a liver function, isn't it?' He replied that it was and that they would keep me posted. I was alarmed and worried. My ex-wife, Pattie, happened to call about twenty minutes later; I told her what was going on and she reminded me that Jesse had jaundice for three weeks at birth. I called Penn back with that information and got somebody who was apparently typing every word I said. That seemed very unusual to me. I didn't hear from the doctors again until mid-afternoon. Dr Mark Batshaw called and said Jesse's condition was worsening, that his blood ammonia was rising, and that he was in trouble. When I asked if I should get on a plane, he said to wait, that they were running another test. He called back an hour and a half later and Jesse's ammonia had doubled to 250 micromoles per deciliter. I told him I was getting on a plane and would be there in the morning.

It's a very helpless feeling knowing your kid is in serious trouble and you are over half a continent away. My plane was delayed out of Tucson but got into Philly at 8 a.m. Arriving at the hospital at eight-thirty, I immediately went to find Jesse. As I entered through the double doors into surgical intensive care I noted a lot of activity in the first room. I waited at the nurse's station for perhaps a minute before announcing who I was. Immediately, Doctors Batshaw and Raper asked to talk to me in a private conference room. They explained that Jesse was on a ventilator and comatose, that his ammonia had peaked at 393 micromoles per deciliter (that's at least ten times a normal reading), and that they were just completing dialysis and had his level down under 70. They explained that he was having a blood-clotting problem and that because he was breathing above the ventilator and hyperventilating, his blood pH was too high. They wanted to induce a deeper coma to allow the ventilator to breath for him. I gave my okay and went in to see my son.

After dressing in scrubs, gloves, and a mask because of the isolation requirement, I tried to see if I could rouse my boy. Not a twitch, nothing. I was very worried, especially when the neurologist expressed her concern at the way his eyes were downcast: 'Not a good sign,' she said. When the intensivist told me that the clotting problem was going to be a real battle, I grew even more concerned. I called and talked to my wife, crying and afraid for Jesse. It was at least as bad as the previous December, only this time something had been done to his liver. I would keep her posted.

They got Jesse's breathing under control and his blood pH returned to normal. The clotting disorder was described as improving and Dr Batshaw returned to Washington, DC, by mid-afternoon. I started to relax, believing Jesse's condition to be improving. My brother and his wife arrived at the hospital around 5:30 p.m. and we went out to dinner. When I returned I found Jesse in a different intensive care ward. As I sat watching his monitors, I noted his oxygen content dropping. The nurse saw me noticing and asked me to wait outside, explaining that the doctors were returning to examine Jesse. At 10:30 p.m., Dr Raper explained to me that Jesse's lungs were failing, that they were unable to oxygenate his blood even on 100 per cent oxygen. I said: 'Whoa, don't you have some sort of artificial lung?' He thought about it for a moment and said yes, that he would need to call in the specialist to see if Jesse was a candidate. I told him to get on it.

I called my wife and told her to get on a plane immediately. At 1 a.m., the specialist, Dr Shapiro, and Dr Raper indicated that Jesse had about a 10 per cent chance of survival on his own and 50 per cent with an artificial lung (an ECMO unit). Hooking it up would involve inserting a catheter into the jugular to get a large enough blood supply. I said, '50 per cent is better than 10. Let's do it.' It seemed to take forever for them even to get the artificial lung ready. Jesse's oxygen level was crashing. At 3 a.m., as they were about to hook Jesse up, Dr Shapiro rushed into the waiting room to tell me that Jesse was in crisis and rushed back to work on him. The next few hours were really tough. I didn't know anything. Anguish, despair, every emotion imaginable went through me. At 5 a.m. Dr Shapiro came to see me and said they had the ECMO working but that they had a major leak, and Dr Raper had his finger on the leak. I quipped that I was a bit of a plumber; maybe that's what they needed. Dr Shapiro returned to work on Jesse and I began to worry about my wife. Hurricane Floyd had made landfall in North Carolina at 3 a.m. and was heading towards Philly.

At 7 a.m. I entered through the double doors into the intensive care area and, after noting four people still working on Jesse and another half-dozen observing, approached the nurses' station to ask them to see if my wife would get in okay. They agreed to check and asked if I would like a chaplain. I'm a pretty tough guy, but it was time for spiritual help. The Christian chaplain, a man a few years younger than me, was called in. At this point I was also trying to contact my family to get emotional support. A hospital staff member was very helpful in that respect.

By mid-morning, six of my siblings and their spouses had arrived. Mickie's plane just got in before they closed the airport and she arrived by taxi in the pouring rain. We weren't able to see Jesse until after noon. Dr Batshaw was stuck on a train disabled by the hurricane. Doctors Raper and Shapiro described Jesse's condition as very grave; that whatever reaction his body was having would have to subside before he could recover. His lungs were severely damaged and if he survived it would be a very lengthy recovery. They had needed to use more than ten units of blood in hooking him up. When we finally got to see Jesse, he was bloated beyond recognition. His eyes were swelled shut and the wax was being extruded out of his ears. The only way we could be sure this was Jesse was by looking at the scar from the battle with his dad on his elbow and the tattoo on his right calf. My siblings were shaken to the core. Mickie touched him ever so gently and lovingly, our hearts nearly breaking.

With the hurricane threatening to close the bridges home, my siblings left by late afternoon. My sister and her husband stayed to take us to dinner and drive us, exhausted, to our hotel. After sleeping for an hour, I arose and felt compelled to return to see Jesse. Leaving Mickie a note, I walked the half-mile back to the hospital in a light rain. Hurricane Floyd had skirted Philly and was heading out to sea. I found Jesse's condition no better. I noted blood in his urine. I thought, 'How can anybody survive this?' I said a quiet goodbye to my son and returned to the hotel at about 11:30 p.m., where I found Mickie preparing to join me. I described Jesse's condition as no different and returned to bed. Mickie went out walking for a couple hours.

The next morning we arrived at Jesse's room by 8 a.m. A new nurse indicated that the doctors wished to speak to us in an hour or so about why they should continue with their efforts. We went to have breakfast at the hospital cafeteria. I knew and told Mickie that we should be prepared for a funeral. She wanted to believe he would get well. Doctors Batshaw and Raper were there when we returned. They told us that Jesse had suffered irreparable brain damage and that his vital organs were all shutting down. They wanted to turn off life support. They left us alone for a few minutes and we collapsed into each other. On their return, I told them that I wanted to bring my family in and have a brief service for Jesse prior to ending his life. Then I told them that they would be doing a complete autopsy to determine why Jesse had died, that this should not have happened. While waiting for my siblings, . moments of anger towards the doctors would sweep over me. I would say to myself, 'No, they couldn't have seen this.' I went so far as to tell Dr Batshaw that I didn't blame them, that I would never file a lawsuit. I was unaware of what they really knew.

Seven of my siblings and their spouses and one of my nieces were present at the brief ceremony for Jesse. Actually, it was more for us at this point. I had all the monitors shut off in his room. Leaning over Jesse, I turned and declared to everyone present that Jesse was a hero. After the chaplain's final prayer, I signalled the doctors. Dr Shapiro shut off the ventilator. After the longest minute of my life, Dr Raper stepped in and I removed my hand from Jesse's chest. Listening with a stethoscope for a moment, Dr Raper said, 'Goodbye, Jesse. We'll figure this out.' There was not a dry eye all around. This kid died about as pure as it gets. I was humbled beyond words. My kid had just shown me what it was really all about. I still feel that way.

I supported these doctors for months, believing that their intent was nearly as pure as Jesse's. Even after the media started to expose the flaws in their work, I continued to support them. I had discovered that federal oversight was woefully inadequate, that many researchers were not reporting adverse reactions, and that industry was influencing the Food and Drug Administration (FDA) into inaction. I decided to attend the Recombinant DNA Advisory Committee (RAC) meeting in December where all the experts were going to discuss my son's death. It wasn't until that three-day meeting Bethesda, Maryland, that I discovered that the experimental intervention my son had undergone was never proven efficacious in humans. I had believed that it was working, based on my conversations with Mark Batshaw, and that is why I defended Penn for so long. But these men could not go in front of their peers at the RAC meeting and say that it was working.

After Penn and the FDA made their presentations on 9 December, I asked for a lunch meeting with the FDA, the National Institutes of Health (NIH), and the doctors from Penn. We touched on many issues and I let them all know that although I had not yet spoken to a lawyer, I would do so in the near future. Too many mistakes had been made and unfortunately, because of our litigious society, legal action was the only way to address these problems.

There is so much more to Jesse's story. I can't help but believe that they will kill this with time and money, as they always seem able to do. Who are 'they'? They are heartless and soulless industry and their lobbyists; they are the politicians and bureaucrats who are more interested in placating industry than in protecting the people; they are physician/researchers who are so blinded in their quest for recognition that they can't even see the dangers any more. Let them apply Jesse's intent to their efforts, and then they'll get it right.

When I wrote 'Jesse's Intent' I was very much a father grieving for his lost son, but my perceptions of what had gone wrong were mostly correct. Looking back, I am even better able to see the flaws in our system. Jesse died because of the money machine that is currently so much a part of medical research. The research scientists, needing funding to continue their work, unwittingly compromised their ethics to keep that money coming. Professional prestige also played an enormous role in influencing the path of this research. My experience in losing Jesse has been very humbling for me. While it was also humbling for the doctors involved, they were still unable openly to admit and apologize for their lapses in judgment before and after Jesse's death.

Doctors Wilson, Batshaw, and Raper must have felt that they had too much to lose by being honest.[2] My first clue that something was amiss came in early November 1999, some six weeks after Jesse's death. One of the principal investigators, Steve Raper, the man who had actually infused Jesse's liver with the viral vector, was in Tucson to help me hike and spread Jesse's ashes on a local mountain top. At a meeting with the University of Arizona researcher who had initially reviewed the OTC study for the government in 1995, I was told in Dr Raper's presence that monkeys had died in the pre-clinical work. The Tucson researcher also expressed his misgivings to me regarding the FDA's oversight efforts and indicated that I should seek out the minutes of the RAC meetings of 1995. Following that meeting, Dr Raper was quick to point out to me that they had changed the original viral vector that had killed monkeys to make it much safer. His explanation at that time satisfied me and I continued my support for their work.

Three weeks later, I discovered the minutes that the University of Arizona researcher had asked me to seek out.[3] As far back as 1995, the FDA and the NIH had been working on a web database to disseminate information on adverse reactions in gene therapy. From the June 1995 minutes of the RAC meeting I learned that the FDA representative had announced that the effort to create a Gene Therapy Information Network had been abandoned. The RAC, indignant because it knew the importance of this database in protecting the participants of research, demanded an explanation. The FDA representative's candid response – 'my superiors answer to industry' – told me volumes.[4] There had been a report in the newspapers at that time that the Schering-Plough corporation had stamped adverse effects in a similar gene transfer study as 'proprietary' and had withheld dissemination of that adverse information.[5] I was incensed at what that meant regarding the oversight of the work. I felt at the time that the Penn researchers had been blindsided by the withholding of that information, and informed them of what I had discovered.

In late November 1999, the head researcher, Dr James Wilson, travelled to my home in Tucson where I met him for the first time, some two months after Jesse's death. He was there to present the findings of Jesse's autopsy. My first question to him, while sitting on my back porch, was, 'What is your financial position in this?' He said that he was an unpaid consultant to the biotech company, Genovo, behind the research effort. Being naive, I accepted his word and continued to support him and his work.

When I decided to attend the Recombinant DNA Advisory Committee meeting in December 1999 Dr Wilson had asked me to fly in a day early to do a morale boost for his 250-person institute at Penn. At first hesitant, I agreed to do it. I had received a phone message the previous Friday from a director within the FDA, Catherine Zoon, and returned her call while waiting for my connecting flight to Philadelphia. I explained to her in no uncertain terms about my discovery of the lapses within the FDA and told her that I would expose the FDA's faulty oversight at the RAC meeting. While at Penn the following day, I was informed by a tearful Dr Wilson that the FDA had just issued a press release blaming his team for Jesse's death. It seemed that I had touched a very sensitive nerve at the FDA. The following day I rose very early and drove to Bethesda. At an FDA press conference, I discovered that the research team had violated the protocol in multiple ways, had not adequately reported serious adverse events in other patients prior to Jesse, and had withheld vital information from the FDA on adverse reactions in animals. The FDA also revealed that Jesse's ammonia level at the time he was infused with the viral vector was well above the limit established as the safe baseline for this study. Realizing that everyone had failed Jesse, I sought legal counsel.

In uncovering the truth of what happened to Jesse, we found some major problems in the informed-consent process. The over-enthusiasm of the clinical investigators led them to paint a misleading picture of safety and efficacy. That enthusiasm blinded them to the ill effects that they were witnessing. They did not communicate those effects to us, or to those responsible for the oversight of their work, notably Penn's research ethics board and the FDA. Some of that blindness appears to have been deliberate. Following Jesse's death, Penn continued misinforming us as to what they knew, telling us only what would keep us on their side.

The Conflict of Interest Committee at Penn had not adequately prevented the conflicts inherent in allowing the lead investigator, James Wilson, and the institution to have a vested financial interest in the clinical trial. Remember that in late November 1999, Dr Wilson had told me that he was an unpaid consultant to the biotech company Genovo. When I testified at a U.S. Senate subcommittee hearing on the problems in gene therapy in February 2000, I met H. Stewart Parker, representative of the biotech lobby and CEO of Targeted Genetics, who also testified. She offered me her condolences for Jesse's death three times. I almost asked her if she had a guilty conscience. She testified that: 'We in the industry were surprised and deeply disturbed to read recent reports of regulatory violations at the Institute of Human Gene Therapy at the University of Pennsylvania. These violations have led to the FDA halting all gene therapy trials underway there. If these violations occurred, this behavior absolutely cannot be tolerated, and penalties should be imposed to the full extent of the law. I am certain that my colleagues in the industry, as well as in gene therapy academia agree with me.' Her next statement, 'As all entrepreneurs must do, I want to get right to the bottom line,'[6] is perhaps closer to the truth than she meant to get.

Her company, Targeted Genetics, bought Dr Wilson's company five months later. He received $13.5 million in stock for his 30 per cent share in the biotech company. So much for being an unpaid consultant.[7] I am certain that Jim Wilson does not see the conflict that the money interests created for him. My experience has told me that, in an effort to protect themselves, a great blindness comes over people who have done serious harm.

The bioethicist who advised the clinical research team, Dr Arthur Caplan, seriously erred when he advised the researchers that they could not obtain informed consent from the parents of dying infants, and should instead test the vector on relatively healthy carriers and partially affected OTC patients. I regard this as a serious violation of the Declaration of Helsinki, since it involved too much risk with no benefit to the research participant. The institutional research ethics board and even the RAC missed this important point.

This same bioethicist was later quoted as saying 'Not only is it sad that Jesse Gelsinger died, there was never a chance that anybody would benefit from these experiments. They are safety studies. They are not therapeutic in goal. If I gave it to you, we would try to see if you died, too, or if you did OK.'[8] I certainly wish that warning had been in the consent form. When Dr Caplan declared that the controversy created by Jesse's death was good for the ethics train, and that 'we [bioethicists] thrive on scandal,'[9] he further demonstrated to me a lack of good judgment. It also turned out that he worked in Dr Wilson's department, effectively making the researcher his boss, another serious conflict. Art Caplan should have seen it coming when he was named as a defendant in our lawsuit.

Interestingly, the nurse who had acted as the informed consent witness when my son was first considered for participation in the clinical trial, and who was the clinical coordinator for his September trip, had resigned her position some ten days prior to Jesse's arrival. Once I realized all the errors that had been committed, I contacted this nurse and discovered that she had resigned because her questions about side effects were not being adequately answered and she was very uneasy about further involvement with the research effort. She had apparently not wanted to make waves, so she just quit. Perhaps if she had expressed her concerns more strongly, someone would have opened their eyes and seen the danger. A more independent advocate may also have helped put the brakes on what occurred.

Apart from the problems with the FDA, we discovered that another federal body, the National Institutes of Health, has a large responsibility in gene transfer research. Only 36 of 970 required adverse event reports were filed with the NIH in the 90 clinical trials using viral vectors similar to the one given to Jesse.[10] Non-compliance with federal guidelines was widespread.

Another area of concern that I uncovered is the peer review process of viable research. In participating in a German documentary that explored why Jesse died, I met a researcher, Günter Cichon, who was dismayed by what occurred, and who had had considerable difficulty in getting a scientific paper published about the severe adverse reactions in rabbits from adenoviral vectors. The paper[11] was finally published in the month Jesse died, after months of undue delay. Dr Wilson was on the editorial review board of the journal[12] in which that paper was published, and was most likely aware of the German data prior to Jesse's death.

These are but a few examples of how our medical research system is rife with conflict of interest. Jesse's case is far more a symptom of a dysfunctional system than an isolated incident of research run amok. A year and a day after Jesse's death, we filed a lawsuit[13] against the three principal investigators, their institutions, and their review boards. I wanted to include the responsible government agencies for their failures but they have immunity. We stuck to our guns and settled our case six weeks later out of court. The quickness of that settlement should tell you how much the other side wanted this to go away. On 10 February 2002 the FDA issued a scathing letter[14] that reads more like an indictment of Dr Wilson, indicating that it was in the final stages of disbarring him from ever again being able to conduct research on human beings. Dr Wilson stepped down as head of the Institute for Human Gene Therapy effective 1 July 2002. He still teaches and is a department chair at the University of Pennsylvania.

For me, a father hoping for the best for my son, the most painful aspect of this whole experience, aside from the loss of Jesse, was the way the doctors and Penn manipulated me after his death. I can understand that Mark Batshaw's misrepresentation of the trial's efficacy was rooted in his enthusiasm to finally secure a viable treatment for doomed infants with OTC. He had dedicated his life to saving these children, but making me a part of their effort to uncover why Jesse died and then not informing me of their earlier failures with the treatment, and using me to help cover their tracks were such egregious acts that I had no choice but to confront them through our lawsuit.

Regardless of the responsible parties' desire for self-preservation, there is a moral obligation on the part of all of us to live up to what Jesse demonstrated: a right heart combined with an unselfish willingness to make this a better world. While many people feel the same way, our system does not reflect that. It paints a false picture of ethical behaviour to disguise what is really going on. We are just research subjects in an enormous marketplace, manipulated into believing the hype and vision of the very ambitious. That ambition is blinding not only the innocent but also those so tied up in the endeavours of modern science that they have no hope of really seeing the right path to the truth. I will always be grateful to Jesse for what he taught me; he was on the right path. We are also very grateful that we live in a society that allowed us to bring a civil suit that brought many of the problems surrounding Jesse's death to light.

Editors' Note: The U.S. Department of Justice's investigation has since resulted in a civil settlement in which the two institutions involved agreed to pay significant penalties totalling over US$1 million to resolve government allegations including false statements to FDA, NIH, and the IRBs charged with oversight of this study. According to the press release, 'reports were submitted that misrepresented the actual clinical findings associated with the study,' and 'the consent form and process did not disclose all anticipated toxicities.' Dr Wilson's clinical and research activity were placed under significant restrictions for at least five years, and Drs Batshaw and Raper for three years. For the Department of Justice press release and links to the settlements, see: http://www.usdoj.gov/usao/pae/News/Pr/2005/feb/UofPSettlement%20release.html. For Paul Gelsinger's comment, see: http://www.circare.org/im/im14Feb2005.htm.

NOTES

1 'Jesse's Intent' was originally published in (2000) 8 Guinea Pig Zero 7. It was reprinted in Robert Helms, ed., *Guinea Pig Zero: An Anthology of the Journal of Human Research Subjects* (New Orleans, LA: Garrett County Press, 2002), 178. It is reprinted here with permission of the publisher.

2 While I have received a personal and private apology from Mark Batshaw, that apology lacked an acknowledgment of responsibility for Jesse's death.

3 James Wilson actually helped steer me to the location of those minutes. One of his right-hand men, Nelson Wivel, hired by Wilson in 1996, had been a director in the NIH office that was responsible for overseeing the Recombinant DNA Advisory Committee. His responsibilities included overseeing the meeting minutes. It should be noted that Nelson Wivel, in his advisory capacity at Penn, knew all the ins and outs of the adverse event reporting requirements to the FDA and the NIH.

4 U.S. Department of Health and Human Services, *National Institutes of Health Recombinant DNA Advisory Committee Minutes of Meeting June 8–9, 1995,* http://www4.od.nih.gov/oba/rac/minutes/6-8-9-95.htm.

5 Sheryl Gay Stolberg, 'New Data Released on Side Effects in Gene Therapy Experiments,' *New York Times,* 20 November 1999, A14.

6 Testimony of H. Stewart Parker before the U.S. Senate Subcommittee on Public Health, http://www.bioventureforum.net/laws/tstm020200.asp.

7 Andrea Knox and Huntly Collins, 'Rival to Buy Local Biotech Pioneer Genovo,' *Philadelphia Inquirer,* 10 August 2000, A01.

8 Michael Matza, 'Lights, Camera, Ethics,' *Philadelphia Inquirer Magazine* 14 May 2000, at 9–13.

9 Huntly Collins, 'Penn Says It Will Alter Gene Therapy Institute,' *Philadelphia Inquirer,* 25 May 2000, A01.

10 Larry Thompson, 'Human Gene Therapy: Harsh Lessons, High Hopes,' *FDA Consumer Magazine* (Sept.–Oct. 2000), http://www.fda.gov/fdac/features/2000/500_gene.html.

11 Günter Cichon et al., 'Intravenous Administration of Recombinant Adenoviruses Causes Thrombocytopenia, Anemia and Erythroblastosis in Rabbits' (1999) 1 J. Gene Med. 360 at 360–71.

12 Editorial Board, *Journal of Gene Medicine,* http://www3.interscience.wiley.com/cgi-bin/jabout/10009391/EditorialBoard.html.

13 *Gelsinger v. University of Pennsylvania*: Complaint filed 18 September 2000, Philadelphia County Court of Common Pleas Trial Division, http://www.sskrplaw.com/links/healthcare2.html.

14 Dennis Baker, Associate Commissioner for Regulatory Affairs, Food and Drug Administration, Department of Health and Human Services to James M. Wilson, MD, PhD, letter dated 8 February 2002, http://www.fda.gov/foi/nooh/Wilson.pdf.

PART ONE

Regulation

2 Questions and Challenges in the Governance of Research Involving Humans: A Canadian Perspective

KATHLEEN CRANLEY GLASS

Most Canadians strongly support the promotion of socially beneficial research. Contemporary health research holds the promise of significant positive developments. But it also clearly poses significant challenges. Issues such as individual, community, and societal risk and personal or institutional conflicts of interest are inadequately addressed in the multi-layered, fragmented, and complex structure of research governance in Canada. Universities and hospitals are confronted with a research funding environment that increasingly relies on private sources of funding and a push to commercialize research results.[1] Yet their researchers receive little assistance in recognizing and managing the conflicts of interest they face, leaving some research subjects inadequately protected.

Maintaining the integrity of Canadian research is not merely a theoretical proposition. Canada is not immune from the difficulties and taint of scandal affecting the history of human research, and requires a solid structure of research governance to protect both those who volunteer to participate and the research enterprise itself. Unfortunately, the current system of governance has serious deficiencies.

The Research Enterprise

Research with humans entails a complex set of activities involving a variety of participants, including public, private, and not-for-profit entities. Pharmaceutical companies operate to research, produce, and market drugs. Hospitals and universities are involved in research and educational activities. Public sector bodies like the national funding agencies – the Canadian Institutes of Health Research (CIHR), the

Social Sciences and Humanities Research Council of Canada (SSHRC), and the Natural Sciences and Engineering Research Council of Canada (NSERC) – fund and promote Canadian researchers. Some federal departments, such as Health Canada and the National Research Council, conduct research on their own account. Disease-based private foundations, patient advocacy groups, and charities provide financial support for research in their areas of interest.

Research must be distinguished from therapy and it requires oversight, given the inherent tension between the primary aims of research and treatment. Where the therapeutic relationship with health professionals is intended to improve the health and well-being of the individual patient, the primary aim of research is to advance knowledge and develop new diagnostic tools and therapies that may benefit patients in the future. Physician investigators may experience tension between their commitments to treatment and commitments to research. Although research subjects often benefit from treatments provided in clinical trials, promotion of the well-being of individuals is not the primary goal of the trial. The primary aim is to answer an established research question. While non-clinical research does not raise the dilemma of the dual role of the physician investigator, there can also be a tension between the inherent drive of researchers to seek answers to their questions and the interests of research subjects.

In Canada, as in other countries, reinforcement of public trust in science has become an important policy objective, especially in the wake of controversies that have to some extent undermined trust in research.[2] There is ample historical evidence to suggest that a researcher's or sponsor's interests in the results of research may at times lead to neglect of the rights and interests of individual research participants.[3] Canada has had its share of research controversies. One of the most notorious scandals involved the scientifically flawed mind-altering experiments by the then world-renowned psychiatrist Dr Ewen Cameron at McGill University's Allan Memorial Hospital in the 1950s.[4] Another instance of questionable practices with human subjects in psychiatric research came to light only recently, with an inquiry into the experimental administration of LSD in Kingston's federal prison for women.[5] The death of a Canadian gene transfer research participant, James Dent, was followed by family allegations that Dent had not been informed that participation involved serious risks, including death, nor was he told that previous U.S. patients in the trial had suffered serious adverse events as a result of participation.[6] The case of Dr Roger Poisson, who falsified research data in breast cancer trials, indicated how potential professional conflicts of interest may induce researchers to commit fraud.[7] More recently, conflicts of interest in research and hiring practices by universities and university-affiliated research institutes,[8] as well as those caused by a publication ban on unanticipated trial risks, have raised questions about the protection of both researchers and their participants.[9]

The Need for Systematic Review of Research

The implementation of research review processes in many countries has developed over time in response to research abuses in which people were exposed to significant risks in the interests of science, often without being informed about it. Gradually, commentators and professional and regulatory bodies came to recognize the need for a systematic means by which to counterbalance the interests of research participants with the inherent desire of researchers to conduct research. This recognition took shape in advocacy for an independent and unbiased evaluation process – a process in which people without a stake in the conduct and outcome of the research would weigh the risks and merits of a given research protocol and evaluate whether research subjects' rights and welfare were sufficiently protected.[10]

Given both the inherent complexity of the process by which scientific evidence is weighed and the financial and professional interests of sponsors and researchers in having their projects proceed, it is essential that conditions for the conduct of research be developed and upheld by people who are independent from the research. Over time, a consensus has developed with respect to the appropriate national and international norms to govern research. Baruch Brody describes the codes and policies governing the ethics of research involving humans as follows:

A clear-cut consensus has emerged in all of these official policies about the conditions of the licitness of research on human subjects. Procedurally, such research needs to be approved in advance by a committee that is independent of the researchers. Substantively, informed, voluntary consent of the subject must be obtained, the research must minimize risks and involve a favorable risk/benefit ratio, there should be an equitable non-exploitative selection of subjects, and the privacy of subjects and the confidentiality of the data must be protected. These substantive standards are rooted in fundamental moral commitments to respect for persons, to beneficence and to justice.[11]

The primary role of the Research Ethics Board (REB) is to help ensure that ethical principles are applied to research involving humans. The review of research by REBs is part of a crucial system of checks and balances, and it should be aimed at protecting those participating in all forms of research. While the focus of a research review process is on safeguarding the rights and well-being of research subjects, the process also reflects a clear recognition of the social importance of the enterprise of research. A sound review process expresses the commitment of society to scientifically valid and ethically sound research, and reinforces public trust in science.[12]

Despite general agreement on the aims and guiding principles for research involving human subjects, however, there is no overarching structure for the governance of research in Canada, and consequently, no process for ensuring that those aims and guiding principles are attained and implemented.

Existing Canadian Governance Mechanisms

Where does the responsibility for research governance lie? Canada has no comprehensive legislation to regulate all research involving humans. Health care research takes place under the legal regime of the common law, or in Quebec, under the *Civil Code*.[13] Laws governing both civil and criminal liability apply, but only to harms after the fact. Additional federal and provincial legislation is applicable concerning a number of issues, including patient/physician privilege, privacy, maintenance of medical records, and capacity to consent.[14] Clinical trials on experimental drugs and devices are regulated federally by the authority of the Health Products and Food Branch of Health Canada.[15] In addition to its own governing regulations, Health Canada participates in the *International Conference on Harmonisation, Choice of Control Group and Related Issues in Clinical Trials* (ICH-E-10), which it applies to trials under Health Canada purview. Trials of pharmaceuticals and devices must also undergo a parallel review process by local institutional REBs. No clinical trial on an experimental drug can proceed unless and until it has passed both Health Canada and REB review. Certain kinds of research in Canada are thus subject to a 'double-review' system. The regulation of research on drugs and devices involves multiple parties influenced by both Canadian and international regulations.

Extra-legal Instruments

Extra-legal instruments also play a very important role in ensuring the ethical conduct of research. A number of codes, guidelines, and policies concerning the conduct of research have been promulgated by various entities, including governmental bodies, funding agencies, professional organizations, and local institutions. Ethics policies often exhort certain behaviour, rather than enforcing it. But even though many of these codes, guidelines, and policies have no formal role in law, in instances where no legal norm exists in a statute or regulation or in case law, the guideline and/or professional norm could have a significant, perhaps even decisive, impact on a judicial decision by assisting courts in setting the accepted standard for judging the actions of an individual or institution in a particular case. Nonetheless, a court as final arbiter of standards may also find that policies or guidelines prescribe inadequate standards, and may formulate more refined norms that meet the legal criteria of reasonableness and diligence.[16]

Guidelines or policies may also be used as the basis for agreements. In the case of Canadian research funding agencies, the *Tri-Council Policy Statement (TCPS)*,[17] was adopted in 1998 as the standard for research undertaken in establishments receiving federal research funding. The agencies have now entered into written memoranda of understanding to assure that all research undertaken within an institution receiving their funds complies with the *TCPS*.

The focus of all of these instruments – legislation, codes of ethics, policies, and guidelines – is the protection of a number of interests, most importantly the physical well-being, inherent dignity, and the integrity of research participants. Other interests include those of investigators in pursuing their professions and the interests of society in increasing knowledge, particularly knowledge bearing on public and individual health.[18]

Government Ethics Structures

The federal government has a number of structures relevant to research ethics, the most prominent of which are the three funding agencies, the CIHR, SSHRC, and NSERC. The CIHR has a Standing

Committee on Ethics within its Governing Council, and an Ethics Office; it also supports the ethics designates who sit on the advisory boards of its institutes. The Interagency Advisory Panel on Research Ethics (PRE) has a stewardship mandate for the *Tri-Council Policy Statement* that includes 'responsibilities for [the policy's] evolution and interpretation, educational implications, and its promotion and implementation.'[19] The National Research Council (NRC) has its own REB, with membership from outside NRC, while Health Canada has an Ethics Division within the Health Policy and Communication Branch. In addition, the federal government established the Canadian Biotechnology Advisory Committee to provide independent advice to a number of federal ministries on the implications of new developments in biotechnology. The federal government and several of the provinces also have privacy commissioners and privacy legislation that affects certain kinds of research.

Non-governmental structures are also involved in the ethics of human research. The National Council on Ethics in Human Research (NCEHR) receives federal funding to advance the protection and promotion of the well-being of research participants and to promote high ethical standards in research. It has provided educational resources for REBs; undertakes site visits, workshops, and training sessions for researchers and REB members; and has produced a number of important studies in the area of research ethics and research review, including a report on accreditation.[20]

Complexity in the Review of Research Studies

A number of circumstances add to the complexity of research review in Canada. For example, research undertaken outside of establishments receiving federal research funds are not bound by the *Tri-Council Policy Statement*. Nor are private REBs, which may therefore use different guidelines to approve research than academic research ethics boards do. In addition, no Canadian REB reviews all research. Which REB will review a proposed protocol or study depends on a number of factors:

- The geographic location of the research is relevant to its review. For multi-site research, there must be REB approval for each site identified for the research.

- The nature of the research may also be a factor. Some institutions have separate REBs for clinical trials, other medical protocols, and for non-health-related research involving human participants.
- Research that will be reviewed by Health Canada must also undergo review and approval by an academic-based REB if it will be conducted at a university teaching hospital site. Most of these institutions receive grants from the three federal funding agencies and are therefore bound by the *Tri-Council Policy Statement*.
- Private REBs generally follow international guidelines, including ICH and the *Declaration of Helsinki*, or the Council on International Organizations of Medical Sciences (CIOMS) research ethics guidelines. They may also voluntarily follow the *Tri-Council Policy Statement*.
- When research funding in Canada comes from an American source, U.S. regulations may apply as well.

These and other factors lead to inconsistencies in review. Decisions regarding approval of the same protocol may vary among REBs, even when they are following the same guidelines or policies. This problem is exacerbated when they follow different guidelines. Such is the case in Canada for placebo controlled trials, where REBs under the *Tri-Council Policy Statement* follow one set of guidelines while Health Canada follows the ICH.[21]

REBs and their host institutions have been reluctant to enter into reciprocity agreements with other REBs.[22] Concerns about potential exposure to legal liability if the same standards of review are not applied at other institutions may motivate such reluctance.[23] Yet such a patchwork of different standards and procedures for the review of clinical trials means that the sponsors of such trials and the researchers who conduct them may incur the added expense of meeting varied requirements for the preparation and submission of study protocols for review.[24]

The Need for Structured Governance of Research in Canada

The current Canadian system of research governance depends primarily upon the REB for oversight. Yet, there is no uniform set of standards that applies across the board to all human subjects research in Canada. We do not have the kind of unifying national regulatory structures found in countries such as France or the United States for most research involving humans. Even with the acceptance of guidelines or policies in Canada, there are no mechanisms for enforcement of the actions of REBs, investigators, or institutions. NCEHR has conducted site visits to institutions on a voluntary basis, but there are no uniform standards for accrediting REBs or their members. At this point, there is no system of national or provincial oversight, and no public oversight of private REBs that act independently or through Contract Research Organizations hired by drug companies. There is no required ethics training for researchers or REB members. In the absence of a national ethics review or advisory body looking at some of the more controversial areas of research, local REBs and their institutions are left to struggle with what may be difficult decisions.[25]

Institutional support for REBs is inconsistent, making monitoring of ongoing research difficult if not impossible for some. Some institutions may be ill-equipped to deal with a rapidly changing research environment, with competition for both private and government research dollars, increasingly complex research, and an ethics review system that relies primarily on the hosts of the research and their REBs to ensure independent ethics review for the protection of human participants.

In the wake of new controversies and published findings of official investigations into historical mishaps there have been a number of recent calls for regulatory reform and overhaul of the research review system.[26] In 1996, the U.S. President's Advisory Commission on Human Radiation Experiments presented a report on radiation experiments conducted between 1944 and 1974 in which people were exposed, sometimes without their knowledge, to various degrees and types of radiation.[27] More recent unexpected deaths of research subjects – one of them in a high-risk gene therapy trial[28] – have added to existing concerns about the adequacy of protections for research subjects. Increased surveillance resulting from these controversies led to the temporary suspension of research activities in some of the most prestigious research institutions in the United States,[29] and concerns have also been expressed in Canada. The Law Commission of Canada commissioned a report on the subject of research governance. Among its findings was that 'Canada's complex, decentralised, multi-sourced arrangements for governing [research with humans] pose major ethical challenges in terms of consistency, transparency and accountability.'[30]

Recurring Research Governance Issues

Given the above discussion, a list of recurring research governance issues might include the following:

- not all research undertaken in Canada is covered by mandatory ethics review;
- REBs are chronically underfunded and rely on volunteers who receive little or no recognition within their institutions for the work they do;
- increased demands for review are being placed on REBs without making corresponding resources available;
- many REBs have reporting structures and membership that create the potential for conflicts of interest within their institutions;
- both REBs and their members lack any sort of accreditation or certification;
- REB members, investigators, and institutional research officers lack education to fulfil their mandates;
- most REBs lack patient or research subject representation;
- there are no standard mechanisms for enforcement of guidelines or policies by REBs or institutions;
- while some institutions have begun to monitor ongoing research, there is a long way to go until all necessary monitoring is in place;
- investigators, hospitals, and academic institutions are under increasing pressure to attract private research funding and push to commercialize results without adequate assistance to recognize and manage the conflicts of interest created by this situation;
- inappropriate reliance by REBs on informed consent of research subjects results in inadequate attention to risk/benefit analysis and inadequate acknowledgment of a physician/researcher's fiduciary duty to subjects who are patients;
- lack of consistent review for multi-site research remains a problem;
- 'forum shopping' for lenient REBs remains a possibility; and
- for many REBs, there is a lack of specialized expertise necessary for review of new forms of research, such as stem cell research, gene transfer trials, research with databases, and research with communities. Neither is there any alternative form of review available, such as a specialized national review committee.

Conclusion

The current system of research governance is fragmented and decentralized, without a consistent, accountable, and transparent system of ethics review. We have yet to establish a comprehensive, uniform set of standards or structure for review that would apply to all research involving humans. There are no viable systems of education, accreditation, or monitoring. Canada needs a governance structure that will ensure independent reporting lines for those responsible for research review, accountability for the actions of those involved in this review, and adequate support for those who are charged to make the system work to protect research participants and ensure the integrity and high quality of Canadian research. In the 2002 Speech from the Throne, the federal government pledged that it would 'work with the provinces to implement a national system for the governance of research involving humans, including national research ethics and standards.'[31] As of this writing, there have been no proposals for such a national system.

NOTES

Kathleen Glass's work on this chapter was funded in part by the Canadian Institutes of Health Research.

1 Sheldon Krimsky, *Science in the Private Interest* (Lanham, MD: Rowman & Littlefield, 2003).
2 Jeffrey M. Drazen, 'Institutions, Contracts, and Academic Freedom' (2002) 34 New Eng. J. Med. 1362 at 1362–3.
3 Kathleen Cranley Glass and Trudo Lemmens, 'Research Involving Humans,' in Timothy Caulfield, Jocelyn Downie, and Colleen Flood, eds., *Canadian Health Law and Policy*, 2nd ed. (Toronto: Butterworths, 2002), 459.
4 Canada, Department of Justice, News Release, 'Background Information – Depatterning at the Allen Memorial Institute' (1992); George Cooper, *Opinion of George Cooper, Q.C., Regarding Canadian Government Funding of the Allen Memorial Institute in the 1950's and 1960's* (Ottawa: Supply and Services Canada, 1986).
5 See Mike Blanchfield, 'LSD Tested on Female Prisoner: Scientists Experimented on Inmates at Kingston's Prison for Women in 1960's,' *Ottawa Citizen*, 28 February 1998, A1; Tracey Tyler, 'Prisoners Used for "Frightening" Tests, New Papers Show,' *Toronto Star*, 18 December 1999; Canada, Correc-

tional Service Canada, News Release, 'Correctional Office of Canada Releases Review Report Prepared by the McGill University Centre for Medicine, Ethics and Law with Respect to the Administration of LSD and ECT at Kingston's Prison for Women in the 1960's' (1998).

6 'In the Service of Science.' CBC Television, The National – The Magazine, 6 March 2000. http://www.cbc.ca/national/magazine/gene/index.html.

7 Charles Weijer, 'Our Bodies, Our Science' (1995) 35:3 The Sciences 41 at 41–5.

8 Glass and Lemmens, 'Research Involving Humans'; David Healy, 'Conflicting Interests in Toronto: Anatomy of a Controversy at the Interface of Academia and Industry' (2002) 45 Perspectives in Biology and Medicine 250.

9 Jon Thompson, Patricia Baird, and Jocelyn Downie, *The Olivieri Report* (Toronto: James Lorimer and Company, 2001).

10 Glass and Lemmens, 'Research Involving Humans.'

11 Baruch A. Brody, *The Ethics of Biomedical Research: An International Perspective* (New York: Oxford University Press, 1998), at 36.

12 Glass and Lemmens, 'Research Involving Humans.'

13 C.C.Q., c. 64.

14 See, e.g., the *Hospital Standards Act*, R.S.S. 1978, c. H-10; *Personal Information Protection and Electronic Documents Act*, R.S.C. 2000, c. 5.

15 *Food and Drug Act*, R.S.C. 1985, c. F-27. This could include the Therapeutic Products Directorate, the Biologics and Genetic Therapies Directorate, or the Medical Devices Directorate, depending on the type of therapeutic agent.

16 Angela Campbell and Kathleen Cranley Glass, 'The Legal Status of Ethics Policies, Codes and Guide-lines in Medical Research and Practice' (2001) 46 McGill L.J. 473 at 473–89.

17 Medical Research Council of Canada, Natural Sciences and Engineering Research Council of Canada, and Social Sciences and Humanities Research Council of Canada, *Tri-Council Policy Statement: Ethical Conduct for Research Involving Humans* (Ottawa: Public Works and Government Services Canada, 1998).

18 Louis L. Jaffe, 'Law as a System of Control,' in Paul A. Freund, ed., *Experimentation with Human Subjects* (New York: George Brazillier, 1970), 197.

19 Canada, Interagency Advisory Panel on Research Ethics (PRE), *Position Paper: Process and Principles for Developing a Canadian Governance System for the Ethical Conduct of Research Involving Humans* (Ottawa, April 2002) at 4, http://www.pre.ethics.gc.ca/english/pdf/Governance_01.pdf.

20 National Council on Ethics in Human Research, *Final Report of the Task Force on Accreditation* (Ottawa: NCEHR, 2002). See also National Council on Ethics in Human Research Task Force on Accreditation, *Options for the Development of an Accreditation System for Human Research Subjects Protection* (Ottawa: NCEHR, 2005).

21 National Placebo Initiative, *Final Report of the National Placebo Working Committee on the Appropriate Use of Placebos in Clinical Trials* (Ottawa: Health Canada and Canadian Institutes of Health Research, 2004).
22 National Council on Ethics in Human Research, *Final Report of the Task Force on Accreditation*.
23 Lorraine E. Ferris, 'Industry-sponsored Pharmaceutical Trials and Research Ethics Boards: Are They Cloaked in Too Much Secrecy?' (2002) 166 Can. Med. Assoc. J. 1279 at 1279–80; Claire Foster, *The Ethics of Medical Research on Humans* (Cambridge: Cambridge University Press, 2001).
24 Joan C. Bevan, 'Towards the Regulation of Research Ethics Boards' (2002) 49 Can. J. Anesth. 900 at 900–6; Tom Beauchamp, 'IOM Report on the System for Protecting Human Research Participants' (2002) 12 Kennedy Institute of Ethics Journal 389.
25 Michael McDonald, ed., *The Governance of Health Research Involving Human Subjects (HRIHS)* (Ottawa: Law Commission of Canada, 2000) http://www.lcc.gc.ca/en/themes/gr/hrish/macdonald/macdonald.pdf.
26 See, e.g., reports by James Bell and Associates for The Office of Extramural Research, *Final Report: Evaluation of NIH Implementation of Section 491 of the Public Health Service Act, Mandating a Program of Protection for Research Subjects*, (Washington, DC: National Institutes of Health, 1998); Office of Inspector General, *Institutional Review Boards: A Time for Reform* (Boston: Department of Health and Human Services, 1997); and National Bioethics Advisory Commission, *Ethical and Policy Issues in Research Involving Human Participants* (Bethesda, MD: National Bioethics Advisory Commission, 2001).
27 President's Advisory Committee on Human Radiation Experiments, *The Human Radiation Experiments: Final Report of the President's Advisory Committee* (New York: Oxford University Press, 1996).
28 Julian Savulescu, 'Harm, Ethics Committees and the Gene Therapy Death' (2001) 27 J. Med. Ethics 148.
29 Ibid.; Harvey Black, 'Research and Human Subjects: Recent Temporary Suspensions, Regulation Initiatives Inject Uncertainty into Study Management' (2000) 14:19 The Scientist 1.
30 MacDonald, ed., *The Governance of Health Research Involving Human Subjects.*
31 Canada, Privy Council Office, Speech from the Throne to Open the Second Session of the Thirty-Seventh Parliament of Canada, 'The Canada We Want' (30 September 2002), http://www.pco-bcp.gc.ca/default.asp?Language=E&Page=InformationResources&sub=sf tddt&doc=sftddt2002_e.htm.

3 Swinging on the Pendulum: Shifting Views of Justice in Human Subjects Research

ANNA MASTROIANNI AND JEFFREY KAHN

Justice has long been one of the central principles in the ethical conduct of research on human subjects. But its application, as reflected in U.S. federal policies pertaining to human subjects research, has undergone a remarkable shift over a relatively short span of time. Understanding this shift is important not only for interpreting claims about justice in human subjects research, but also for assessing the status and adequacy of policies for protecting subjects.

In the 1970s, these policies emphasized the protection of human subjects from the risks of harm in research, and justice was seen as part of this protection. Since the early 1990s, however, justice as applied in research ethics has emphasized the need to ensure access to the potential benefits research has to offer. That such a dramatic shift could occur so quickly is extraordinary, especially in light of the understanding, coalescing over the same period, that subjects have an inadequate understanding of the research in which they are participating and are inadequately protected by existing practices and policies. The tension between these developments offers an important lesson for research protection as the context of human subject research becomes more complex. Our goal here is to attempt to understand how the pendulum has swung from protection to access, where in its arc we are, and where we should be.

Justice in the Belmont Era: Protection from Exploitation

The development of human subject protection policy in the United States was driven by a history of exploitation of subjects, most notably by research on 'vulnerable' subject populations that came to light between the mid-1960s and the early 1970s. The landmark examples were the Willowbrook State School hepatitis vaccine research on institutionalized children;[1] the Jewish Chronic Disease Hospital cancer research, involving the injection of cancer cells into elderly nursing-home residents;[2] and the so-called Tuskegee Syphilis Study,[3] which had been underway for decades but was exposed to an appalled nation in 1972.[4]

Those examples contributed to a sense that human subjects research in the United States permitted scandalous practices – inadequate attempts to inform subjects about research and obtain their consent, exploitive recruitment strategies, the use of vulnerable subject populations, and a willingness to expose subjects to significant risk without any potential for direct medical benefit. Further, there was a sense that the risks and benefits of research were split unfairly: the risks were borne by subjects, while the benefits accrued to others.

The early history of U.S. research ethics policy thus focused on the risks rather than the benefits of research, and on preventing subjects from being exposed to unacceptable or exploitive levels of risk, particularly without the prospect of offsetting direct medical benefits. The Belmont Report, issued by the National Commission for the Protection of Human Subjects of Biomedical and Behavioral Research in 1978, identified justice as requiring the fair distribution of the burdens and benefits of research in subject selection and recruitment; in practice, however, justice was interpreted as requiring the prevention of any further exploitation of vulnerable groups.[5] The emphasis was realized through the promulgation of research policies that staked much on protection and that singled out particular groups – prisoners, children, pregnant women, and foetuses – for additional protections.

Prisoners were deemed vulnerable because of the nature of their living environment. Adequate informed consent, it was believed, was not possible when subjects lived in a setting that constrained the autonomy on which the concept of informed consent is based. This view actually ran counter to information collected by the National Commission, which found in interviews with prisoners who participated in research that the prisoners wanted to be enrolled in studies, and were highly motivated research subjects, for a variety of reasons – among them the opportunity to earn a few extra dollars, the perks that might come with research participation, access to more frequent and potentially improved health care, and a belief that participating in research offered a way for them to make a contribution to society. Most interesting was the finding that it was not the least powerful and arguably most vulnerable prisoners who participated in research, but the most powerful.[6] Prisoners often viewed research as an opportunity to be seized rather than a hazard to be avoided; they apparently did not worry that anyone was taking advantage of them. Even so, policies were promulgated, and remain in place today, that made it impossible to perform research on prison populations unless the research either offers a prospect of direct medical benefit to the individual subjects themselves, as in clinical trials for HIV infection, or aims at understanding or improving the prison environment, so that it would potentially benefit prison populations generally.

Children were deemed vulnerable because of similar concerns about informed consent and the potential for taking advantage of their reliance on others. Such concerns were vividly illustrated in the infamous Willowbrook case, where hepatitis vaccine research was performed on institutionalized, mentally retarded children whose parents seemed to have little choice but to agree to their children's participation – thereby selecting the most vulnerable from among the potential pool of children. The rules developed to prevent this sort of exploitation limited research in which children could participate to studies involving either minimal risk or direct medical benefit.

Pregnant women and foetuses were deemed especially vulnerable and deserving of protection. Influenced by the abortion debate and memories of thalidomide, policy makers excluded pregnant women from research that carried risk of harm, to protect them and their foetuses. The implementation of this policy was expanded in practice to include not only pregnant women but also women of childbearing capacity, both to prevent unwitting risk to foetuses and to protect the future health of the women. This practice represented the logical conclusion of a regulatory culture and process that emphasized the protection of subjects from risk as paramount.

From Protection to Access

The research regulatory culture that emphasized protection from risk in the 1970s began to change in the late 1980s and early 1990s. Due to a growing belief that research increasingly offered real benefits, the application of justice in research began to emphasize the fair distribution of the benefits of research instead of its risks. Advocacy groups, particularly those representing the interests of people with AIDS and women's health groups, argued this view to great effect before Congress and elsewhere. The thrust of their position was that fairness demands not only protection from the risks of research, but increasingly the opportunity for inclusion in research. The emphasis on justice as protection was shifting to justice as access.

The HIV/AIDS advocacy community was at the forefront of making the case for justice as access. As the first clinical trials for AZT were being undertaken, groups like ACT-UP organized rallies protesting the limited enrolments in them. At a time when subjects were sharing their research medication with friends to spread around whatever potential benefit could be had from these drug trials, protestors were marching in large cities across the country carrying placards proclaiming 'Clinical trials are health care too!'[7] Such a sentiment, conflating research participation with medical care, represented not merely a shift in emphasis but a total reversal of the ethics of research.

Through the late 1970s and 1980s, there was a growing sense that cutting edge therapy could be found in research participation, particularly for cancer, where the best therapeutic outcomes were thought to be in research protocols, and where standard treatment modalities were largely viewed as less effective. It was certainly true that the benefits from the major investments in biomedical research were being realized and applied. The problem was that those benefits were most likely to be realized by the groups represented in the subject populations – largely, although not exclusively, adult Caucasian males. Whatever the complex of reasons for excluding women, racial and ethnic minorities, and children from research participation, the policy was largely predicated on protection from harm and exploitation. But as advocates began to point out, such policies, while they may have prevented harm and exploitation, also prevented benefit – resulting, as one commentator claimed, in a climate that protected some groups to death.[8] Exclusion denies access to the benefits of research at two levels – first to the individuals who may themselves receive the direct medical benefit of research participation, and more notably to the groups from which the subjects come.

There are numerous examples of the research system's failure to provide equitable benefits to women. Among the most notable is the United States Physicians Study, a longitudinal study that assessed the effectiveness of low dose aspirin for preventing heart attacks.[9] It yielded strong evidence of success, but could not be applied outside the research population, comprised exclusively of men, because women are not merely smaller versions of men. Similarly, children are not merely smaller versions of adults, and racial and ethnic groups may differ from each other in disease pathology, drug response, and the like.

The realization that policy and practice had emphasized protection and a denial of the real and perceived benefits of research pushed the pendulum of research policy towards recognizing the importance of access to the benefits of biomedical research, by means of policies requiring inclusion in research set against a background of protection. In 1994, less than twenty years after the first federal policies on research protections were promulgated, the U.S. National Institutes of Health (NIH) issued the first policy requiring inclusion of particular groups in research – the Guideline on Inclusion of Women and Minorities in Research.[10] This guideline represents an unprecedented sea change in thinking about the ethics of research on human subjects.

Implementing Justice in Policy

The implementation of the 1994 NIH guideline flipped the presumption about research participation from exclusion to inclusion. Researchers were and are now required to include representative populations of women and minorities in their protocols unless there are special reasons for excluding them. It would make no sense, for example, to include women in a clinical trial testing a new drug for prostate cancer, nor would it be reasonable to conduct research on conditions in racial or ethnic groups in which those conditions are not found.

Policy on the participation of children in research is following a similar path, driven by similar arguments. In an effort to protect them, children have been excluded from research that carried greater than minimal risk unless the research also had the potential to provide direct medical benefit to the subjects. Thus U.S. federal regulations[11] bar the participation of children in Phase I drug trials, which are used to assess the safety of new drugs before their approval. But excluding children from such research has meant there is limited information about the safety of drugs in paediatric populations. This information has instead been pieced together after the drugs are approved and marketed for adults: children have received drug doses based only on the most general calculations of their size relative to the adults for whom drugs are approved, and ongoing clinical experience of paediatricians who have begun to try the drugs on children.

Recent directions from both the NIH and the U.S. Food and Drug Administration are changing the presumption from exclusion to inclusion, and requiring a special justification to exclude children.[12] The change in approach has not been completely achieved, however. Reversing the presumption about participation has resulted in a policy that reflects the tension between ensuring access to the benefits of research and protecting subjects from research harms. The dictates of Subpart D, as currently written, do not easily coexist with a policy of inclusion. It appears that the long-standing commitments to protection will be weakened as part of the trend towards ensuring access to the benefits of research.

Changes in the rhetoric of health policy are further evidence of the emphasis on access to the benefits of research, reaching to the highest levels of the U.S. government. Richard Klausner, while director of the National Cancer Institute, testified before Congress in 1998 about the need for large increases in the overall NIH budget (which were eventually granted), arguing that substantial additional resources were required 'to ensure that all people who wish to participate in a clinical trial are able to do so.'[13] The comment both presupposes that there is a real benefit to be had by the subjects of clinical research and reflects a remarkable commitment to universal access to research participation, particularly in a country where there is no similar commitment concerning basic health care.

Klausner's commitment has now been realized in policy, at least for those who have health insurance or are eligible for Medicare. In 1999, United Healthcare, one of the largest managed care organizations in the country, became the first third-party payer to agree to pay the costs associated with their subscribers' participation in cancer clinical trials.[14] The decision was hailed as a major step in removing one of the substantial barriers to participation in clinical trials generally, since the policy of most health insurers has been to deny payment for the costs of clinical trial participation on the grounds that the treatment rendered is experimental. Whether the change in policy is a function of a changed view of the benefits of research participation, a response to the demands of its customers, or a commitment to supporting the research that yields the clinical advances on which health care depends, it certainly delivers a message to patients: if your insurance company thinks research is worth paying for, it must be worth participating in. Not long after the decision was announced, then-President Bill Clinton directed the Medicare payment system to ensure that

Medicare recipients would enjoy similar access to clinical trial participation, leaving it to policy makers to determine the conditions under which patients would be eligible for such a benefit. The current rule provides Medicare coverage for participation in Phase II or later trials.[15] This theme even became part of the rhetoric of the 2000 presidential campaign, when presidential candidate Al Gore incorporated a reference to access to research participation in his standard stump speech on health care issues.[16]

The final piece of evidence that the pendulum has swung fully from protection to access is the waiver of informed consent in research in emergency settings, written into U.S. federal regulations in 1996.[17] The waiver is the ultimate endorsement of an emphasis on the benefits of research, since it suggests that research participation is so beneficial to individuals and society that we must guarantee access even for those unable to consent. With this step, we have now backed away from the cornerstone concept of informed consent, dating back to the Nuremberg era, in the protection of research subjects.

A New Era in the Protection of Human Subjects?

What are the implications for research oversight of the swing from protection to access? The protection of the rights and interests of research subjects is rightly the pre-eminent concern in research oversight, but how do we ensure that protection is adequately balanced against access? There is ample evidence that even in an environment stressing protection there are serious shortcomings in the process of informed consent,[18] and subjects are persistently confused about the distinction between research and clinical care[19] and the benefits they stand to realize by participating in research.[20] An overemphasis on the benefits of research participation can undermine the reality that research inherently carries risk and very often holds no benefits to the subject.

It is a confusing time to be a subject – or to be thinking about becoming one. The media presents stories about the need for more research and research funding alongside reports of serious harms to subjects in research trials. The death of Jesse Gelsinger in a gene transfer study at the University of Pennsylvania resulted in a swirl of reportage, congressional hearings, university investigations, and new restrictions and reporting policies for gene transfer research.[21] The *Seattle Times* reported on alleged conflicts of interest and failures to obtain informed consent in two clinical trials in which some subjects died unexpectedly, both at Seattle's Fred Hutchinson Cancer Research Center.[22] The *Los Angeles Times* ran a story on 'seven deadly drugs' that were fast-tracked to approval by the Food and Drug Administration (FDA) and subsequently withdrawn from the market after they were discovered to have serious side effects, sometimes leading to death.[23] Moreover, the FDA asked for an additional US$36 million in fiscal year 2002 to increase its 'emphasis on high-risk trials, such as those enrolling vulnerable populations (mentally impaired and pediatric populations, for example ...'[24] How do we reconcile these divergent messages to subjects, investigators, Institutional Review Boards (IRBs), and institutions, and properly balance the requirements of justice in research? If we fail to answer this question adequately, we risk a serious erosion of trust in the research enterprise.

In Pursuit of Trust: From Compliance to Conscience

Accountability for balancing protection and access falls to those at every level in the conduct of research: the physicians who refer their patients to investigators, the investigators themselves, the IRBs that oversee research, and the institutions where research is performed. Policy making does not occur in a vacuum; regulatory and spending decisions respond to the perceived needs and expressed desires of the public. Without trust from the public, there can be no research, as there will be no research subjects willing to participate and no willingness on the part of the public to support research with tax dollars. Research should be understood as a privilege not to be presumed or exploited, but earned through building and maintaining the public trust. This requires a careful balancing of access and protection.

The efficacy and consistency of oversight systems to protect human subjects continue to be an area of study and criticism. Recent reports, investigations, and legal actions have been directed primarily at the institutions and IRBs that serve as the linchpins of research oversight, concluding that they do not work as well as they should, or as we would hope, in protecting individual subjects from research harm.[25] In one such investigation, the U.S. Food and Drug Administration and the Office of Human Research Protections (OHRP) suspended research at a prestigious research institution after the death of a research subject, for lapses in regulatory compliance and oversight.[26] At least one high-level state court has admonished researchers, research institutions, and policy makers for their failure to adequately protect children in research.[27] In addition, numerous publications have uncovered institutions and researchers with financial conflicts of interest that might have the potential to harm or mislead research subjects or otherwise affect the quality of the research.[28] Announcements by the Department of Health and Human Service's Office of Human Research Protections as well as the National Institutes of Health focus on such conflicts of interest in research, actions which are, at base, efforts to secure public trust by ensuring in part that investigators are not biased in ways that may lead them to overlook the protection of subjects.[29]

These critical assessments have spawned a series of governmental and institutional responses formulated to ensure policy compliance and protect research subjects from harm. Such responses have included implementation of IRB accreditation processes, educational mandates for investigators, and recommendations for mandated disclosures of potential conflicts of interest.[30] In practice, however, it appears that, regardless of their original intent to protect subjects, these strategies, in conjunction with federal enforcement and private liability actions, have instead fostered a culture of institutional caution and an overemphasis on compliance. Researchers, and even the director of the OHRP, have complained about overzealous implementation of policies by research institutions and their IRBs (e.g., consent forms that number in the hundreds of pages, reporting of adverse events determined to be unrelated to studies, IRB meeting minutes with volumes of supporting documentation), actions that do not contribute to the safety of research subjects and at the same time slow down the review process.[31] Social scientists complain loudly about institutional misapplication of biomedical research requirements to their studies.[32]

Overall, there has been an increasing sense that this overemphasis on paperwork and other minutiae of compliance may lead to even less reflection on why the rules are important. The former director of the OHRP, Greg Koski, made the point well when he said that the research community needed to move 'beyond the culture of compliance ... to a culture of conscience and responsibility.'[33]

Research as Partnership

At the same time, an approach to research has been emerging that may counter such overly strict interpretation of the rules. This approach considers research a partnership among all the participants in the process, altering the relationship between institutions, researchers, and the subjects of research. Rather than policies and practices being dictated by those overseeing research, practices are discussed, negotiated, and eventually agreed upon by those involved in it. Community groups, their representatives, and the individuals who belong to communities are taking a greater role in the planning, design, recruitment, and approach to the sharing of research benefits. Research conceived of as partnership is different, and this shift can lead to changes in practice and policy that can be agreed upon and endorsed at all stages of research, turning the subjects of research into fuller partners in the research enterprise. In short, this is a movement towards a shared decision-making model. Recent rhetoric from the federal government, such as the OHRP slogan, 'Doing it well ... together,' supports this trend, as does the increasing use of the term 'research participant' in lieu of 'research subject,' when it appropriately describes the relationship.

Community research models, including efforts by research institutions to work more closely with communities, community partnerships for health, consultation with groups and communities affected by genetic research, and increasing recognition of non-physical harms in community research, all point to the trend towards treating research more as a partnership. Research as partnership changes the dynamic of protection and access in new ways by creating a more equitable relationship among researchers and subjects/participants. In so doing, the partnership model supports both greater (and more appropriate) protections as well as assuring greater access to the benefits deemed appropriate by those most directly affected by the research. This helps to balance the swing between protection and access.

Such commitment to partnership has implications for the entire process of research. There can be partnerships among those who do research, those who oversee it, the institutions at which it is done, and the relationships created with the communities that were asked to participate in the research. Ultimately, this increases trust. Real partnership and adequate protections will never be achieved unless there is a trust relationship among the researchers, their institutions, research participants, and the groups that they represent. As always, that includes trust in investigators, trust in institutions, and trust in the processes for those oversight protections.

These commitments must not come solely in the form of pronouncements from institutional officials. Such pronouncements can lead to an increasing sense that rules and requirements act more like obstacles than improvements to the research environment. For many researchers, they translate into a culture of resentment rather than a culture of commitment. What is required is a change in the culture in which research is carried out. Until these changes occur, we will find it difficult to achieve real partnership in a commitment to the ethics of human subject research. Instead, we will live with an undercurrent of resentment for the rules imposed, and find it increasingly difficult to foster the trust that is so crucial to successful and ethically acceptable research on human subjects.

With the renewed interest in protection – whether it be real or on paper – in the current research climate, the pendulum may have swung as far as it can towards an emphasis on benefits. Increasing policy attention to conflicts of interest, reporting, and regulatory oversight of the research environment seem to be a sign that the pendulum has begun its swing back towards an emphasis on protection. But paperwork requirements are not enough. What remains to be seen is how far the pendulum will go, and whether we have the tools to control it.

NOTES

Originally published in substantial part as Anna Mastroianni and Jeffrey Kahn, 'Swinging on the Pendulum: Shifting Views of Justice in Human Subject Research' (2001) 31 Hastings Center Report 21.

1 The Willowbrook study involved children who were institutionalized at a residence for mentally retarded children. Parents who were applying to place their children in the institution were sometimes told that no space was available except in the research wing, whose residents were enrolled in the vaccine study. When the study was made public in a newspaper exposé, concerns were raised around the enrolment of institutionalized mentally retarded children in research that did not seem to offer potential benefit to them, as well as about the adequacy of parental consent.
2 Research in the Jewish Chronic Disease Hospital involved a study by researchers from a prominent cancer treatment centre that recruited subjects from a long-term care facility for the purpose of determining immune response when cancer cells are introduced into the body. It required injecting elderly subjects who did not have cancer with cancer cells taken from other patients. Disclosure of this research led to an investigation by New York state authorities and subsequent administrative actions. The issues

raised were familiar: recruitment of an easily exploited subject population, no potential for direct medical benefit to the subjects, and inadequacy of informed consent.

3 The infamous so-called Tuskegee Syphilis Study, with its well-known abuses of African-American men, deceitfully recruited these men into a study of the natural history of syphilis by promises of treatment. Again, the concerns centred on the exploitation of subjects, no potential for direct medical benefit to them, and inadequate (or lack of) informed consent.

4 James Jones, *Bad Blood* (New York: Free Press, 1993).

5 U.S., National Commission for the Protection of Human Subjects of Bio-medical and Behavioral Research, *The Belmont Report: Ethical Principles and Guidelines for the Protection of Human Subjects of Research* (Bethesda, MD: Department of Health, Education, and Welfare, 1978).

6 U.S., National Commission for the Protection of Human Subjects of Bio-medical and Behavioral Research, *Report and Recommendations: Research Involving Prisoners* (Bethesda, MD: Department of Health, Education, and Welfare, 1976); Victor Cohn, 'Prisoner Test Ban Opposed,' *Washington Post*, 14 March 1976, A7.

7 Randy Shilts, *And the Band Played On: Politics, People, and the AIDS Epidemic* (New York: St Martin's Press, 1987).

8 Alta Charo, 'Protecting Us to Death: Women, Pregnancy, and Clinical Research Trials' (1993) 38 Saint Louis U.L.J. 135.

9 JoAnn E. Manson et al., 'Aspirin in the Primary Prevention of Angina Pectoris in a Randomized Trial of United States Physicians' (1990) 89 Am. J. Med. 772.

10 *NIH Guidelines on the Inclusion of Women and Minorities as Subjects in Clinical Research*, 59 Fed. Reg. 14,508 (1994).

11 45 C.F.R. § 46.401–9 [Subpart D].

12 U.S., National Institutes of Health, *NIH Policy and Guidelines on the Inclusion of Children as Participants in Research Involving Human Subjects* (6 March 1998), http://www.nih.gov/grants/guide/1998/98.03.06.

13 Robert Pear, 'Medical Research to Get More Money from Government,' *New York Times*, 3 January 1998, A1.

14 Gina Kolata and Kurt Eichenwald, 'Insurers Come in from the Cold on Cancer,' *New York Times*, 19 December 1999, §4, 6.

15 Robert Pear, 'Clinton to order Medicare to Pay New Costs,' *New York Times*, 7 June 2000, A24. The resulting final Medicare coverage decision can be found at http://www.cms.hhs.gov/coverage/8d.asp.

16 James Dao, 'Gore Urges Doubling of Funds in War Against Cancer,' *New York Times*, 2 June 2000, A18.

17 *Waiver of Informed Consent Requirements in Certain Emergency Research*, 61 Fed. Reg. 51,531 (1996); *Protection of Human Subjects: Informed Consent*, 61 Fed. Reg. 51,498 (1996).

18 Advisory Committee on Human Radiation Experiments, *The Human Radiation Experiments* (New York: Oxford University Press, 1996), at 439–58 [*Human Radiation Experiments*]; Clarence H. Braddock, 'Advancing the Cause of Informed Consent: Moving from Disclosure to Understanding' (1998) 105 Am. J. Med. 354; Eric D. Kodish et al., 'Informed Consent in the Children's Cancer Group: Results of Preliminary Research' (1988) 82 Cancer 2467.

19 *Human Radiation Experiments*, at 459–81; Nancy E. Kass *et al.*, 'Trust: The Fragile Foundation of Contemporary Biomedical Research' (1989) 19 Hastings Center Report 25.

20 Paul S. Appelbaum, Loren H. Roth, and Charles W. Lidz, 'The Therapeutic Misconception: Informed Consent in Psychiatric Research' (1982) 5 Int'l J. L. & Psychiatry 319; Christopher Daugherty et al., 'Perceptions of Cancer Patients and Their Physicians Involved in Phase I Trials' (1995) 13 J. Clinical Oncology 1062.

21 Daniel S. Greenberg, 'Stricter Regulation Proposed for U.S. Gene Therapy Trials' (2000) 255 Lancet 1977 at 1977.

22 Duff Wilson and David Heath, 'Uninformed Consent,' *Seattle Times*, 11–15 March 2001.

23 David Willman, 'How a New Policy Led to Seven Deadly Drugs,' *Los Angeles Times*, 20 December 2000, A1.

24 James G. Dickinson, 'When FDA Doesn't Want Preemption' Medical Device & Diagnostic Industry (February 2001) 42, http://www.devicelink.com/mddi/archive/01/02/005.html.

25 Daniel D. Federman, Kathi E. Hanna, and Laura Lyman Rodriguez, eds., *Responsible Research: A Systems Approach to Protecting Research Participants* (Washington, DC: National Academy Press, 2002); Institute of Medicine, *Preserving Public Trust: Accreditation and Human Research Participant Protection Programs* (Washington, DC: National Academy Press, 2001); Rita McWilliams et al., 'Problematic Variation in Local Institutional Review of a Multicenter Genetic Epidemiology Study' (2003) 290 J. Am. Med. Assoc. 360.

26 Lawrence K. Altman, 'F.D.A. Faults Johns Hopkins Over Process in Fatal Study,' *New York Times*, 3 July 2001, A12; James Glanz, 'Agency Eases Research Ban at University,' *New York Times*, 24 July 2001, A1.

27 *Grimes v. Kennedy Krieger Institute*, 782 A.2d 807 (Md. 2001).

28 See, e.g., Robert Matthews, 'Researchers' Links with Biomed Industry Lead

to Bias in Clinical Trials,' *New Scientist* 177:2380 (1 February 2003) 8; Patricia Baird, Jocelyn Downie, and Jon Thompson, 'Clinical Trials and Industry' (2002) 297 Science 2211; David Korn, 'Conflicts of Interest in Biomedical Research' (2000) 284 J. Am. Med. Assoc. 2234; Frank Davidoff et al., 'Sponsorship, Authorship, and Accountability' (2001) 345 New Eng. J. Med. 825.

29 Jeffrey Brainard, 'U.S. Seeks Power to Fine Universities over Human Research' (2000) 46:39 Chronicle of Higher Education A38.

30 See Association for the Accreditation of Human Research Protection Programs (AAHRPP) at http://www.aahrpp.org/www.aspx; U.S., National Institutes of Health, *Required Education in the Protection of Human Research Participants* (5 June 2000, revised 25 August 2000), http://grants.nih.gov/grants/guide/notice-files/NOT-OD-00-039.html; AAMC Task Force on Financial Conflicts of Interest in Clinical Research, 'Protecting Subjects, Preserving Trust, Promoting Progress I: Policy and Guidelines for the Oversight of Individual Financial Interests in Human Subjects Research' (2003) 78 Acad. Med. 225; AAMC Task Force on Financial Conflicts of Interest in Clinical Research, 'Protecting Subjects, Preserving Trust, Promoting Progress II: Principles and Recommendations for Oversight of an Institution's Financial Interests in Human Subjects Research' (2003) 78 Acad. Med. 237; Nils Hasselmo, 'Individual and Institutional Conflict of Interest: Policy Review by Research Universities in the United States' (2002) 8 Sci. & Engineering Ethics 421.

31 'Researchers Over-Implementing Safety Regs; OHRP to Help Community Find Proper Limits' *Medical Research Law and Policy Report* 2:22 (19 November 2003) 801.

32 Constance F. Citro, Daniel R. Ilgen, and Cora B. Marrett, eds., *Protecting Participants and Facilitating Social and Behavioral Sciences Research* (Washington, DC: National Academy Press, 2003).

33 Philip J. Hilts, 'New Voluntary Standards are Proposed for Experiments on People,' *New York Times*, 29 September 2000, A14.

PART TWO

Conflict of Interest

4 The Ethical and Legal Foundations of Scientific 'Conflict of Interest'

SHELDON KRIMSKY

'Conflict of interest' is embedded in many areas of public ethics. Certain enactments named for their ethical content, such as the U.S. *Ethics in Government Act*, have sections devoted to 'conflict of interest,' and the legal community, government officials, financial organizations, and many news organizations have strict guidelines on such conflict. Yet the term is rather new to the scientific and medical research communities. Prior to 1980 little public attention was given to scientists with competing interests in their research. The first medical journal to introduce a conflict of interest disclosure requirement was the *New England Journal of Medicine* in 1984, followed a year later by the *Journal of the American Medical Association*.[1]

One might ask whether conflicts of interest among scientists should be treated differently than they are in other professions. Why, moreover, did the concern about conflicts of interest arise so much later among scientists, compared to public policy and law? This chapter explores the ethical and legal foundations of conflict of interest (COI) in the sciences and asks whether COI among scientists, in contrast to other professions, represents an ethical problem.

Science and Ethics

Conflict of interest in science and medicine has been defined as a set of conditions in which professional judgment concerning a primary interest (i.e., integrity of research) tends to be adversely influenced by a secondary interest (i.e., financial gain).[2] There are two possible explanations for why the issue of conflict of interest arose late among the scientific professions: (1) scientists were believed to operate within a normative system that mitigates any concerns about such conflict, and (2) considerable public trust afforded to scientists, including clinical investigators, eclipsed any potential societal concerns about competing interests.

Science is a self-governing system, subdivided into professional societies, journals, and communication networks, referred to as the 'invisible colleges' that define the shared areas of study, outlets of publication, and collaboration of similarly trained individuals.[3] Its normative structure, emphasizing the importance of scepticism, replication, and empirical verifiability, according to some observers, makes any other interests scientists may have irrelevant to the mission of science. Only one set of interests can lead to success within the profession – the unfettered commitment to methodological rigour and the pursuit of verifiable knowledge.

Throughout the nineteenth and much of the twentieth centuries, with the exception of Nazi science, which is generally viewed as an aberration, the ethics of science was uniquely tied to its epistemology, insulating it from public oversight. It was not until the 1970s that the bubble of normative insularity of science was burst, specifically for clinical trials and human experiments generally. Scientists using human subjects are in a fundamental conflict of interest that is inherent to the process. As researcher, the primary concern of the scientist is to determine the truth about the effectiveness and efficacy of a treatment. The focus has to be on the observance of sound methodology, honest data gathering, and statistical rigour. If too many subjects are dropped from a trial, the results may not be publishable in the most competitive journals.

As a clinician, however, the researcher has a responsibility (as expressed by the Hippocratic Oath) to do no harm and to try to help a sick patient get better. In their effort to balance these goals, clinical researchers sometimes fail to disclose all the risks facing the subject, or fail to stop the trial for a subject who is having adverse reactions. Alternatively, they may make a premature leap from animal studies to human trials in their enthusiasm to reach a positive outcome for a drug before their competitors do. In the wake of highly publicized cases where the concerns of human subjects were discounted in favour of a researcher's professional interests, legislation or regulation emanating from funding agencies focusing on the protection of human subjects was adopted in the United States, Canada, and other countries with advanced centres of biomedical research.

The long tradition of trust in science was rooted in the myth of the scientist as a selfless investigator of universal truths. As scientists proved their utility to civilization in the eighteenth and nineteenth centuries, some philosophers and scientists alike began to think of science as also providing insights into the moral order of the universe – an idea with roots in Greek philosophy. As J.H. Randall noted in his classic work, *The Making of the Modern Mind,* 'The Order of Nature contained an order of natural moral law as well, to be discovered and followed like any other rational principles of the Newtonian worldmachine.'[4] Philosophers of science who believed that there was a parallel between the formal structure of science and that of ethics proposed a theory of ethics based upon a deductive nomological system comparable to mathematical physics.[5] The aspiration of developing a system of ethics derived from natural law or modelled on the mathematical sciences met its demise concurrently with the refutation of logical positivism as the foundation of philosophy.

Another view held by some sociologists of science and natural scientists writing *qua* humanists is that the culture of science has its own ethical system, which serves as a model for other sectors of society. Jacob Bronowski popularized the view that 'science has humanized our values,'[6] while Robert Merton introduced the normative structure of the social system of scientific organizations, which he observed in the early twentieth century.[7]

The conditions under which scientists and government officials, including judges, carry out their fiduciary responsibilities may be quite different. In addition, the normative constraints on science and government and the lines of accountability are distinct. Conflicts of interest in science and government are not necessarily rooted in a similar ethical matrix or based on a comparable legal foundation. In fact, one might justifiably question whether COI in science can be grounded in *any* ethical matrix. The discourse over COI in science might just be about political correctness. We can, however, object to conflicts of interest in science and medicine on grounds other than ethical ones. If there *is* an ethical basis for addressing conflicts of interest among academic scientists, we need to consider the ethical principle (or principles) on which it rests. I shall begin this inquiry by asking the following questions: What factors establish COI as an ethical concern in public affairs? Do those factors apply to scientific COI? If not, do other considerations apply to scientists?

COI in Government

Government employees are stewards of the public's policies, its land, laws, and regulations. Federal officials who use their positions to gain personal financial benefit are in conflict with their fiduciary role as stewards of public resources. In this sense they are trustees of the public's properties, regulations, and its legal traditions. COI *behaviour* (financially self-serving decision making) is a violation of the ethical principle that government employees should not use their positions for personal gain. Generally, we cannot know whether a decision of a public official was made out of self-interest or whether that self-interest and public interest happen to coincide. Why not regulate or punish *only* the behaviour that violates the ethical principle?

Andrew Stark, in his book *Conflict of Interest in American Public Life,* provides a three-stage anatomy of conflict of interest.[8] The *antecedent acts* (stage 1) are factors that condition the state of mind of an individual towards partiality, thereby compromising the potential of that individual from exercising his or her responsibility to foster public rather than private or personal interests. Examples are government employees accepting gifts, paid dinners, and the like. The *states of mind* (stage 2) represents the affected sentiments, dispositions, proclivities, or affinities conditioned by the antecedent acts. Thus, a politician who accepts a substantial campaign contribution from an individual may be more inclined to favour that individual's special business needs in legislative decisions than if no contribution were given.

The final stage represents the outcome behaviour or *behaviour of partiality* (stage 3) of the public official or those actions taken by that individual (decision behaviour) arising from a state of mind affected by the antecedent acts. The outcome behaviour could result in self-aggrandizement or in rewarding friends at the expense of the general public interest.

If public conflict-of-interest law were directed only at stage 3, the behaviour of partiality, this would have several implications. First, a person could be found guilty of conflict of interest only if it could be proved that his or her behaviour resulted from gifts, favours, or mutually self-serving relationships. We cannot infer the disposition or intention of the public employee from the outcome of a policy or regulatory decision. It is difficult to characterize a person's state of mind. Consider the case where a U.S. president issued a pardon to a person living outside the United States who was charged with a felony and who never stood trial. Funds contributed to the president's campaign can be traced to the alleged felon's immediate family. How would one show that there is a link between the gifts, the President's state of mind, and the decision to issue a pardon?

The third implication of focusing exclusively on outcome behaviour in COI law is that it would have little prophylactic effect. Most of the damage is already done by the time the legal processes kick off. Only a small number of cases would be prosecuted, since the burden of demonstrating violations would be high.

As Stark notes, 'because we cannot prevent officials from mentally taking notice of their own interests, we prohibit the act of holding certain kinds of interests in the first place.'[9] Therefore, the law operates on the public health model of 'primary prevention.' Public employees are required to be free of any conditions that may dispose them to act in a way that elevates self-interest (particularly financial self-interest) over public interest.

In public health 'primary prevention' means eliminating the exposure. In COI terminology, 'primary prevention' means 'avoiding the appearance of conflict of interest.' The best of our journalists operate on a preventative principle by not accepting lunch, gifts, or drinks from a person they interview. The ethical principle may be stated as follows: To protect the public's confidence in a free and independent press, journalists must comport themselves in such a way that avoids even the appearance that they could gain a financial benefit from the slant or context of a story or the way in which they present an individual.

Does the stewardship frame apply to scientists? In fact, scientists do have some stewardship functions. A great majority of the grants scientists receive in academic research are from public funds. Scientists are obligated to use the funds according to the provisions of the grant. They are expected to publish the results of their research in the open literature. If an American scientist makes a commercially useful discovery from his/her publicly funded grant, then under the *Bayh-Dole Act* (1980), the U.S. government transfers all intellectual property rights to the discovery to the researcher and his/her institution. This is a case where public investment is turned into private wealth, indicating a limited stewardship role of the scientist over the grant income.

The stewardship frame does not fit well with the self-image of university scientists, who place a high premium on academic freedom and independence. It is also not consistent with federal policies, which have created incentives for faculty to partner with for-profit companies and to start their own businesses. In other words, the U.S. government provides incentives for academic scientists to hold conflicts of interest. The government has reconciled these tensions by requiring disclosure and COI management of federal grant recipients at their institutions.

Another reason the U.S. government does not embrace the steward-ship frame for COIs is that it would place a high burden on federal agencies for waiving a COI. Moreover, because the university is the legal recipient of the federal grant, it would have to address institutional conflicts of interest, a decision that the U.S. government has deferred.

Under the 1972 *Federal Advisory Committee Act* (FACA), agency advisory committees are explicitly forbidden to be inappropriately influenced by special interests, and its members must comply with federal conflict of interest laws designed to protect the government process from 'actual or apparent conflicts of interest.'

Two rules guide the U.S. federal advisory committee structure on conflicts of interest.[10] The first states that no person with a substantial conflict of interest can serve on a federal advisory committee. A federal employee may not 'participat[e] personally and substantially in an official capacity in any particular matter in which, to his knowledge, he or any other person ... has a financial interest if the particular matter will have a direct and predictable effect on that interest.'[11] However, the second rule holds that the first rule can be waived.

In a study of Food and Drug Administration (FDA) advisory committees covering more than a year and a half, *USA Today*'s investigative journalists found that there were 803 waivers for conflicts of interests in 1,620 member appearances, or about 50 per cent.[12]

Scientists are not stewards of public law or natural resources, certainly not in the way public employees or elected officials are. As recipients of public grants, it might be argued that academic scientists have stewardship of public funds and thus their relationship to those funds must be clear of conflicts of interest. This is not a popular argument, and it was not used to justify the Guidelines on Conflict of Interest issued by the National Science Foundation and the Public Health Service. The title of the Public Health Service Guidelines on conflict of interest is 'Objectivity in Research.'[13] Thus, managing COIs among scientists was viewed as promoting scientific integrity, not protecting public law, regulations, or property from being compromised by personal interests.

Disclosure of Interests

While 'stewardship ethics' does not seem applicable to academic science, another ethical response to scientific COI, one which has gained moderate acceptance in recent years, is transparency. The argument for scientists to disclose their conflicts of interest might be framed as follows. Scientists are expected to abide by the canons of their discipline even as they hold other interests, such as financial interests, in the subject matter of their research. The disclosure of one's financial interests (patents, equity holdings, honoraria) is deemed a responsibility because it allows peer reviewers, editors, and readers to look at published studies with additional scepticism.

Organized scepticism, one of the four Mertonian norms,[14] plays a central part in the scientific culture. A good scientific paper will discuss possible methodological limitations of a study and sources of bias. In many fields, it is considered the responsibility of the author to invoke a self-referential scepticism. Disclosure of one's financial interest in the subject matter of a paper falls into that tradition of barring all reasonable biases.

An author's financial disclosure might suggest to reviewers or readers that they consider how hidden biases related to the revealed interest might have entered the study. Also, disclosure allows editors to decide whether the conflicts are so egregious that the paper should not be published in their journal.

Disclosure also provides another social value. When an author's commercial affiliations are not cited in the publication of a paper but are learned after a controversy erupts, it makes it appear that the scientist has something to hide, even if he/she does not. In other words, with the lack of transparency of affiliation, public trust in science is diminished.[15]

Is disclosure a sufficient ethical response to scientific COI? Disclosures considered under COI policies or guidelines when scientists submit a paper for publication, testify before Congress, are recipients of a federal grant, or serve in an advisory capacity include whether the scientist:

- is a stockholder in a company that may benefit from research, a review, or an editorial;
- is a paid expert witness in litigation;
- receives honoraria from companies;
- is a patent holder;
- is a principal in a company that funds his/her research;
- serves as a paid member of a scientific advisory board or board of directors of a company.

The application to clinical trials of the informed consent ethical framework has recently come under debate. There are two streams of thinking here. One view is that COI is inherently unethical in clinical trials because it breaks the trust relationship between patient and physician. The second view holds that COI is not inherently unethical but must be part of the well-established informed consent process. Thus far, informed consent has focused on the nature of the medical intervention, including risks and benefits to the subject. Introducing COI into the informed consent process is viewed by some as a marked departure from the ethics of patient care.

In the case of the tragic death of Jesse Gelsinger in September 1999, the young man was not fully advised of the conflicts of interest involved in his experimental gene therapy treatment. During the investigations following Gelsinger's death, it was learned that the director of the University of Pennsylvania's Institute for Human Gene Therapy, James Wilson, founded a biotechnology company called Genovo, Inc. Both he and the University of Pennsylvania (Penn) had equity stakes in the company, which had invested in the genetically altered virus used in the gene therapy experiment. Wilson and one of his colleagues had also been awarded patents on certain aspects of the procedure. Genovo at the time contributed a fifth of the $25 million annual budget of Penn's gene therapy institute and in return had exclusive rights over any commercial products. The informed consent documents made no mention of the specific financial relationships involving the clinical investigator, the university, and the company. The eleven-page consent form Gelsinger signed had one sentence that stated that the investigators and the University of Pennsylvania had a financial interest in a successful outcome. When Genovo was sold to a larger company, James Wilson had stock options reported to be worth $13.5 million; the university's stock was valued at $1.4 million.[16] According to the report in the *Washington Post*, 'numerous internal U. Penn. documents reveal that university officials had extensive discussions about the possible dangers of such financial entanglements.'[17]

The Gelsinger family filed a wrongful death lawsuit against the university, which was eventually settled out of court for an undisclosed sum of money. One of the plaintiff's allegations in the suit was that the clinical investigator overseeing his trial had a conflict of interest that was not adequately disclosed prior to Jesse Gelsinger's involvement. They argued that the financial interests in conjunction with other undisclosed or downplayed risks might have altered the family's risk benefit estimate before entering the trial and saved young Gelsinger's life. After Penn settled with the Gelsinger family, the university administration announced new restrictions on faculty involved in drug studies when they have equity in companies sponsoring the research.

In the aftermath of the Gelsinger case, the Department of Health and Human Services (DHHS), under the leadership of Secretary Donna Shalala, held hearings on whether the financial interests of clinical investigators should be listed on informed consent documents given to prospective candidates for clinical trials. In a draft guidance document DHHS suggested that researchers involved in clinical trials disclose any financial interests they have to Institutional Review Boards that monitor other ethical issues and possibly to the patients deciding whether to participate as human subjects. Leading scientific and medical associations, including the Federation of American Societies of Experimental Biology (FASEB) and the American Association of Medical Colleges (AAMC), opposed the idea of a guidance document for clinical trials, arguing that it over-regulates medical research without contributing to the safety of patients.

Millions of Americans participated in more than 40,000 clinical trials in 2002, about 4,000 of which were supported by the National Institutes of Health (NIH). Research scientists and the companies sponsoring those trials were concerned that the additional disclosure requirements with no direct bearing on the safety or benefits of the trials would create unnecessary impediments to attracting human volunteers. On the other hand, the decision to become a human volunteer in a medical experiment can be one of the most important choices a person can make. Why should a prospective volunteer not know everything of relevance to the trust relationship they are asked to develop with the clinical investigator?

Conflict of interest in clinical trials has become an ethical issue because of the perceived fiduciary responsibility of the clinical investigator to disclose all relevant information to the human subject. This legal responsibility was upheld by the California Supreme Court in the case of the MO-Cells, cells taken from John Moore during his surgery without his informed consent.[18]

Consequentialist Ethics of COI

Does anything intrinsically unethical occur when a scientist engages in research in which he or she has a commercial interest? To answer affirmatively we would have to demonstrate that such a condition would violate the scientist's fiduciary responsibility to some person or persons, or that there is an inherent conflict between any of those relationships and the scientists' goal or mission *qua* scientist. With the exception of human subjects research, there is no compelling argument here. I can find no inherent reason why scientists cannot pursue the truth and still participate in the commercialization of that knowledge. The two activities do not appear to be logically or conceptually in conflict. But the context and consequences of scientific COI may be ethically significant. Does possessing a commercial interest in the subject matter of one's research have other, unintended effects?

In his book *Real Science*, John Ziman addresses the question of the significance of 'disinterestedness' in ensuring the objectivity of science.[19] He observes that in the current climate of commercial science, 'what cannot be denied is that the academic norm of disinterestedness no longer operates.'[20] While Ziman asserts that we can no longer assume 'disinterestedness' as a norm in this period of 'post-academic science,' 'the real question is whether their [scientists'] interests are so influential and systematic that they turn science into their unwitting tool.'[21] In other words, will the loss of 'disinterestedness' result in the demise of objectivity?

Ziman distinguishes between two concepts of objectivity. He defines cognitive objectivity as an epistemic concept that refers to the existence of physical entities and their properties and that is independent of what we may know about them. Cognitive objectivity is attained when we tap into the properties of the 'objective world,' that segment of the physical universe that exists independent of our thought processes.

Social objectivity is defined by Ziman as the perception that the knowledge process is not biased by the personal self-interest of the knower. Despite the loss of 'disinterestedness' in science, Ziman believes that cognitive objectivity can be protected. 'The production of objective knowledge thus depends less on genuine personal "disinterestedness" than on the effective operation of other norms, especially the norms of communalism, universalism and scepticism. So long as post-academic science abides by these norms, its long term cognitive objectivity is not in serious doubt.'[22]

I dwell on Ziman's work because he provides an important context for understanding society's ethical and legal response to scientific COI. Cognitive objectivity is the verifiable and dependable knowledge science seeks. If that knowledge is not threatened by the loss of disinterestedness, then society's response to COI may be decidedly different than if it were. And while social objectivity (the public's perception of objectivity) may be important, its loss does not, in itself, affect the quality of certifiable knowledge – the published research in our peer-reviewed journals.

How can we determine whether cognitive objectivity is preserved in post-academic science? In contrast to other methods of fixing belief, science is considered to be self-correcting. It is generally understood that, in the long run, systematic bias and errors in science will eventually be disclosed and corrected. However, the time period for self-corrections in science to take place can be quite protracted. It took about 1800 years before Galileo corrected Aristotle's laws of motion. While errors or bias in modern science may not have to wait that long to be discovered, they can be very damaging even for short periods. Witness the work of Sir Cyril Burt on twin studies and IQ: Burt's results influenced cognitive psychologists and educational theorists for decades before it was discovered to be a fraud.[23] The faith we have in the self-corrective nature of science must be viewed against the effects of biased studies in fields like biomedicine, toxicology and material science. Within this context we may ask whether multi-vested science is distorted by a conflict of interest effect. In Ziman's words, will the loss of disinterestedness affect cognitive objectivity? A relatively new body of research can help us answer this question.

In the consequentialist framework, the ethics of COI is viewed in terms of whether holding a conflicting interest correlates with one of the transgressions in science. The burden is to demonstrate a link between possessing a COI and some level of scientific misconduct or bias. The generally accepted transgressions in science include the following:

- scientific fraud;
- failure to give informed consent;
- wanton endangerment of human or animal subjects;
- plagiarism; and
- systematic bias.

Borderline ethical issues include:

- unwillingness to share scientific data/information; and
- participation in ghost writing.

A COI can be said to be an ethical issue in science if it disposes a scientist to commit an ethical transgression – that is, if it increases the probability that the scientist will violate his/her professional responsibility. If COI does not affect the professional responsibility of scientists, then perhaps efforts taken towards managing COI have, as suggested above, more to do with political correctness than with righting an ethical wrong.

In 1996 Les Rothenberg and I published a study which showed that lead authors of articles published in fourteen highly rated journals had a 34 per cent likelihood of having a financial interest in the subject matter of the publication. *Nature Magazine* wrote an editorial stating that:

> It comes at no surprise to find ... that about one third of a group of life scientists working in the biotechnology rich state of Massachusetts had financial interests in work they published in academic journals in 1992. The work published makes no claim that the undeclared interests led to any fraud, deception or bias in presentation, and until there is evidence that there are serious risks of such malpractice, this journal will persist in its stubborn belief that research as we publish it is indeed research, not business.[24]

Five years later, *Nature* reversed itself and decided it would introduce conflict of interest requirements for authors.[25] In its editorial announcing the change of policy *Nature* wrote, 'there is suggestive evidence in the literature that publication practice in biomedical research has been influenced by the commercial interests of authors.'[26]

What do we know about the relationship between possessing a financial interest and bias? Is there a funding effect in science? If there is evidence that the private funding of science produces conclusions biased towards the interests of the sponsor, then we have a genuine cause for treating COI as an ethical problem. The first set of systematic studies that looked at whether there was an association between the source of funding and the outcome of a study was centred on the drug industry.

One of the most elegant and influential studies demonstrating an association between funding source and outcome was published in 1998 in the *New England Journal of Medicine* by a Canadian research team at the University of Toronto.[27]

This study began with the question of whether there was an association between authors' published positions on the safety of certain drugs and their financial relationships with the pharmaceutical industry. The authors focused their study on a class of drugs called calcium channel antagonists, which are used to treat hypertension. Their choice was based on the fact that the medical community debated the safety of these drugs. The researchers performed a natural experiment to investigate whether the existing divisions among researchers over the drug's safety could be accounted for by funding sources, whether, that is, medical researchers were financially connected to the pharmaceutical industry, and whether those affiliations explained their conclusions.

First, the authors identified medical journal articles on calcium channel blockers (CCBs, also known as channel antagonists) published between 10 March 1995 and 30 September 1996. Each article (and its author) was classified as being supportive, neutral, or critical with respect to these drugs. Second, the authors were sent questionnaires which queried whether they had received funding in the past five years from companies that manufacture either CCBs or products that compete with them. The investigators ended up with seventy articles (five reports of original research, thirty-two review articles, and thirty-three letters to the editor). From the seventy articles, eighty-nine authors were assigned a classification (supportive, neutral, or critical). Completed questionnaires about author financial interests were received from sixty-nine authors. The study results showed that an overwhelming number of the supportive authors (96 per cent) had financial relationships with manufacturers of CCBs, while only 37 per cent of the critical authors and 60 per cent of the neutral authors had such relationships. The authors of the *New England Journal of Medicine* study wrote that 'our results demonstrate a strong association between authors' published positions on the safety of calcium-channel antagonists and their financial relationships with pharmaceutical manufacturers.'[28]

Other studies confirm a funding effect for randomized drug trials,[29] economic analyses of new drugs used in oncology,[30] and research on nicotine's effect on human cognitive performance.[31]

Marcia Angell, former editor of the *New England Journal of Medicine*, commented that it was her impression that 'papers submitted by authors with financial conflicts of interest were far more likely to be biased in both design and interpretation.'[32] Angell's impression was validated by findings that appeared in the *Journal of the American Association* from a meta-type analysis on the 'extent, impact, and management of financial conflicts of interest in biomedical research.'[33] Beginning with a screening of 1,664 original research articles, the authors culled 144 that were potentially eligible for their analysis and ended up with 37 studies that met their criteria. One of the questions the authors pursued in their study was whether there was a funding effect in biomedical research. Eleven of the studies they reviewed found that industry-sponsored research yielded pro-industry outcomes. The authors concluded:

> Although only 37 articles met [our] inclusion criteria, evidence suggests that the financial ties that intertwine industry, investigators, and academic institutions can influence the research process. Strong and consistent evidence shows that industry-sponsored research tends to draw pro-industry conclusions. By combining data from articles examining 1140 studies, we found that industry-sponsored studies were significantly more likely to reach conclusions that were favourable to the sponsor than were nonindustry studies.[34]

There are perhaps a dozen or so studies that confirm the funding effect in science for clinical drug trials. The effect has also been confirmed for tobacco research[35] and postulated but not rigorously analysed for toxicological studies of industrial chemicals,[36] nutrition research,[37] and policy studies.[38] Notwithstanding these results, there is no evidence that COI is correlated with scientific fraud or other serious ethical violations. Moreover, it is difficult to assess how generalized or pervasive the funding effect is. To reach the conclusion that research studies authored by scientists with commercial interests in the subject matter is inherently unethical (on the basis of a few dozen selected studies) because of a potential funding effect is neither defensible nor practical. There is, after all, over $2 billion in private research and development (R&D) funding going to U.S. universities (about 7 per cent of the total R&D budget in academia). To make the case that privately funded research fails the objectivity test and therefore is unethical would require a vast study of studies in a variety of disciplines as well as replication of results.

A recent survey reported in the journal *Nature* of several thousand U.S. scientists begins to provide some of the answers. Early and mid-career scientists were asked to respond anonymously to sixteen questions on their research behaviour. One of the questions scientists were asked was whether they have changed the design, methodology, or results of a study in response to pressure from a funding source; 20.6 per cent of the mid-career scientists and 9.5 per cent of the early career scientists answered affirmatively.[39]

Several sectors, such as privately funded tobacco research, have been targeted as untrustworthy. As a consequence, some universities have refused to accept tobacco money for research or other purposes. In areas where the funding effect in science has not been confirmed, a consequentialist ethic for managing conflicts of interest (where assessing moral significance is predicated on their consequences to science) may not apply. There is, however, another ethical framework which has been incorporated into legal doctrine and applied to other sectors to prevent or minimize COI.

Integrity of Science as an Ethical Norm

Protecting the integrity of scientific enterprise is embedded in the scientific ethos. Organized scepticism, objectivity, disinterestedness, correcting mistakes, punishing scientific misconduct, peer review, and institutional review boards are all part of the system the scientific community has established to protect the integrity of the scientific enterprise. One can argue that a scientific discipline replete with conflicts of interest is likely to lose its integrity in the eyes of the general public because it appears to be accountable to interests other than the pursuit of truth. In Ziman's terms, even if science's cognitive objectivity is protected, the social objectivity of science will be threatened.

> In the eyes of the public, the major virtue of academic scientists and their institutions is that, even when they do disagree, they can be trusted to present what they know 'without fear or favour.' Whether or not this high level of credibility is really justified, it is what gives science its authority in society at large. Without it, not only would the scientific enterprise lose much of its public support: many of the established conventions of a pluralistic, democratic society would be seriously threatened.[40]

There is a quantity-quality relationship. As a field of science becomes increasingly commercialized, the quality of the science and the public's confidence in it suffers. Just think of cigarette science, or the studies funded by the lead or the chemical industry. The goal behind these industry-funded research agendas is to manufacture uncertainty for the purpose of derailing or postponing regulation. If the protection of scientific integrity is a societal goal and conflict of interest is an obstacle to reaching that goal, then COI should be viewed as an ethical issue. Moreover, preventing or minimizing COI becomes an ethical imperative.

We try to prevent COI in legal procedures because it erodes the goal of a fair trial. Federal judges cannot own a single stock in a company that is a litigant in their courtroom. It would be inconceivable for society to accept a judge's declaration that, in deference to transparency, he would disclose that he was sentencing a convicted felon to serve his sentence in a for-profit prison in which he, the judge, has equity interests. The courts are exclusively funded by public sources; universities and professors receive funding from public and private sources. We cannot apply the same standards. But there are certain conditions where the integrity of research is so critical to public trust that a response is warranted.

What can be done to restore the integrity of academic science and medicine at a time when turning corporate and blurring the boundaries between non-profit and for-profit are in such favour? We should perhaps begin by harkening back to the principles on which universities are founded. We should consider the importance of protecting those principles from erosion and compromise for the sake of amassing larger institutional budgets and providing more earning potential for select faculty members. I have proposed several principles:

- the roles of those who produce knowledge in academia and those stakeholders who have a financial interest in that knowledge should be kept separate and distinct;
- the roles of those who have a fiduciary responsibility to care for patients while enlisting them as research subjects and those who have a financial stake in the specific pharmaceuticals, therapies, or other products, clinical trials, or facilities contributing to patient care should be kept separate and distinct; and
- the roles of those who assess therapies, drugs, toxic substances, or consumer products and those who have a financial stake in the success or failure of those products should be kept separate and distinct.[41]

The ethical foundations needed for protecting the integrity of science demand measures that go beyond the mere disclosure of interests.[42] If disclosure were the only solution, scientists would be viewed as simply other stakeholders in an arena of private interests vying for epistemological hegemony. The ethical principles – as ideals – would require that certain relationships in academia be prohibited. The legal foundations, however, remain uncertain. Currently, the law has little to offer on the question of preventing a clinical investigator from having a financial conflict of interest in therapies while caring for patients or supervising clinical trials. Universities have become the self-managers of COI both among their own faculty and for their own institution. There are no legal sanctions for transgressing a norm, because there are no established legal norms. In other areas of public ethics, the laws are more explicit. In the United States, the roles of financial auditors and accountants have been under more scrutiny since the Enron affair. New rules have separated auditing from other financial dealings. Legal separation of conflicting roles, however, has not reached the scientific community, perhaps because scientists, unlike lawyers, politicians, and accountants, are still viewed as adhering to a standard of virtue that renders them immune from compromise by their involvement with commercial interests. Recent scientific evidence reveals a quite different picture.

NOTES

1 Marcia Angell and Jerome P. Kassirer, 'Editorials and Conflicts of Interest,' Editorial (1996) 335 New Eng. J. Med. 1055; Catherine D. DeAngelis, Phil B. Fontanarosa, and Annette Flanagin, 'Reporting Financial Conflicts of Interest and Relationships between Investigators and Research Sponsors,' Editorial (2001) 286 J. Am. Med. Ass'n 89.
2 Dennis F. Thompson, 'Understanding Financial Conflicts of Interest' (1993) 329 New Eng. J. Med. 573.
3 Diana Crane, Invisible Colleges: Diffusion of Knowledge in Scientific Communities (Chicago: University of Chicago Press, 1972) at 35.
4 John Herman Randall, The Making of the Modern Mind (Boston: Houghton Mifflin, 1976).
5 Henry Margenau, Ethics and Science (Princeton, NJ: D. Van Nostrand, 1964) at 138.
6 Jacob Bronowski, Science and Human Values (New York: Harper & Row, 1965) at 70.
7 Robert K. Merton, Social Theory and Social Structure (New York: Free Press, 1949).

8 Andrew Stark, *Conflict of Interest in American Public Life* (Cambridge, MA: Harvard University Press, 2000).

9 Ibid. at 123.

10 18 U.S.C. §208(a)–(b).

11 5 C.F.R. § 2640.103(a).

12 Dennis Cauchon, 'FDA Advisors Tied to Industry,' *USA Today* (25 September 2000) 1A at 10A.

13 *Objectivity in Research*, 42 C.F.R. § 50.601–7 (1995).

14 The norms of science cited by Robert Merton are communalism (or communism), disinterestedness, organized scepticism, and universalism. See Merton, *Social Theory and Social Structure* at 552–61.

15 One editor reported removing a previously published paper from all citation indexes after he learned the author failed to report a conflicting interest. Griffith Edwards, 'Addictions Decision to Withdraw a Published Paper from Citation on the Grounds of Undisclosed Conflict of Interest' (2002) 97 Addiction 756.

16 Jennifer Washburn, 'Informed Consent,' *Washington Post*, 20 December 2001, W16.

17 Ibid. at W23.

18 *Moore v. The Regents of the University of California*, 793 P.2d 479 (Cal. 1990).

19 John Ziman, *Real Science* (Cambridge: Cambridge University Press, 2000) at 162.

20 Ibid. at 174.

21 Ibid. at 171.

22 Ibid. at 174.

23 Richard C. Lewontin, Steven Rose, and Leon J. Kamin, *Not in Our Genes* (New York: Pantheon Books, 1984) at 107.

24 'Avoid Financial "Correctness,"' Editorial (1997) 385 Nature 469.

25 'Declaration of Financial Interests,' Editorial (2000) 412 Nature 751.

26 Ibid.

27 Henry T. Stelfox et al., 'Conflict of Interest in the Debate Over Calcium-Channel Antagonists' (1998) 338 New Eng. J. Med. 101.

28 Ibid. at 101.

29 Lise L. Kjaergaard and Bodil Als-Nielsen, 'Association Between Competing Interests and Authors' Conclusions: Epidemiological Study of Randomized Clinical Trials Published in BMJ' (2002) 325 Brit. Med. J. 249; John Yaphe et al., 'The Association Between Funding by Commercialized Interests and Study Outcome in Randomized Controlled Drug Trials' (2001) 18 Family Practice 565.

30 Mark Friedberg et al., 'Evaluation of Conflict of Interest in Economic Ana-

lyses of New Drugs Used in Oncology' (1999) 282 J. Am. Med. Ass'n 1453; Sheldon Krimsky, 'Conflict of Interest and Cost-Effectiveness Analysis' (1999) 282 J. Am. Med. Ass'n 1474.

31 Christina Turner and George J. Spilich, 'Research into Smoking or Nicotine and Human Cognitive Performance: Does the Source of Funding Make a Difference?' (1997) 92 Addiction 1423.

32 Marcia Angell, Testimony (Plenary Presentation at the Conference on Human Subject Protection and Financial Conflicts of Interest, Department of Health and Human Services, National Institutes of Health, Bethesda, MD., 15–16 August 2000) at 36, http://www.aspe.hhs.gov/sp/coi/8-16.htm.

33 Justin E. Bekelman, Yan Li, and Cary P. Gross, 'Scope and Impact of Financial Conflicts of Interest in Biomedical Research' (2003) 289 J. Am. Med. Ass'n 454.

34 Ibid. at 463.

35 Deborah E. Barnes and Lisa A. Bero, 'Why Review Articles on the Health Effects of Passive Smoking Reach Different Conclusions' (1998) 279 J. Am. Med. Ass'n 1566; Deborah E. Barnes and Lisa A. Bero, 'Industry-Funded Research and Conflict of Interest: An Analysis of Research Sponsored by the Tobacco Industry Through the Center for Indoor Air Research' (1996) 21 J. Health Pol'y. 516.

36 Sheldon Rampton and John Stauber, *Trust Us, We're Experts* (New York: Putnam, 2001); Marvin S. Legator, 'Industry Pressures on Scientific Investigators' (1998) 4 Int'l J. Occup'l & Envtl. Health 133.

37 Marion Nestle, *Food Politics* (Berkeley: University of California Press, 2003) at 118.

38 'Safeguards at Risk: John Graham and Corporate America's Back Door to the Bush White House' (Washington, DC: Public Citizen, 2001).

39 Brian C. Martinson, Melissa S. Anderson, and Raymond deVries.'Scientists Bahaving Badly, *Nature* (9 June 2005) 435:737–8.

40 Ziman, *Real Science* at 175.

41 Sheldon Krimsky, *Science in the Private Interest: Has the Lure of Profits Corrupted Biomedical Research?* (Lanham, MD: Rowman & Littlefield, 2003) at 227.

42 Lisa A. Bero, 'Accepting Commercial Sponsorship: Disclosure Helps – But Is not a Panacea' (1999) 319 Brit. Med. J. 653.

5 Self-Censorship

JAMES ROBERT BROWN

The ideals of science are easier to describe precisely and endorse cheerfully than they are to observe scrupulously. Open and free inquiry, shared results, an absence of taboo subjects, and so on, are part of the package. We often hear that 'political correctness' is undermining these laudable aims by hampering research into sensitive subjects, such as race or gender and cognition. Scientists who pursue such topics claim to be unfairly hounded on non-scientific grounds, and so other researchers, not wanting to feel similar unpleasant pressures, censor themselves and pursue less socially sensitive topics.

I am quite sceptical about this alleged attack on free inquiry. But if there is a grain of truth to this scenario, it is as nothing when compared to the amount of self-censorship brought on by commercial factors. Indeed, to be concerned with political correctness while ignoring commercial intrusions betrays a colossal ignorance of what is genuinely important to both science and society.

Much has been written about the negative influence of commercial interests on science. There is a variety of ways in which science can be debased. Self-censorship is one of these, though it is little explored. One of the reasons for this lack of investigation is that, unlike many other aspects of commercialization, self-censorship is almost wholly non-quantitative, and its extent is thus very difficult to measure. I must, therefore, content myself in this brief article with a more anecdotal approach.

Before discussing self-censorship explicitly, let me briefly review some of the corrupting influences that the increase in commercialization has brought, starting with the evaluation of patentable products.

With no other information at hand, we would naturally expect that the results of any test could go either way. That is, when a random drug X produced by company A is compared with drug Y produced by company B, we would expect X to prove better than Y about half of the time in treating some specific medical condition. These may indeed be the actual results of serious scientific study – but they are not the results that get published. Remarkably, when the study in question is funded by one of the pharmaceutical companies, the sponsor's drug invariably does better. Richard Davidson, for instance, found that in his study of 107 published papers that compared rival drugs, the product produced by the sponsor of the research was found to be superior in every single case.[1] It seems that Lady Luck smiles on sponsors. People with this sort of persistent luck in the lotteries, however, are usually investigated for fraud.

The Davidson study is typical; there are many coming to similar conclusions, though not quite so dramatically. For instance, Friedberg et al.[2] found that only 5 per cent of published reports on new drugs that were sponsored by the developing company gave unfavourable assessments. By contrast, 38 per cent of published reports were unfavourable when the investigation of the same drugs was sponsored by an independent source.

Stelfox et al.[3] studied seventy articles on calcium-channel blockers. These drugs are used to treat high blood pressure. The articles in question were judged as favourable, neutral, or critical. The finding was that 96 per cent of the authors of favourable articles had financial ties with a manufacturer of calcium-channel blockers; 60 per cent of the authors of neutral articles had such ties; and only 37 per cent of authors of unfavourable articles had financial ties. Incidentally, in only two of the seventy published articles was the financial connection revealed.

With these cases in mind, we rightly become worried about who is funding the research and what effects that funding is having, effects that are far from the spirit of ideal science. The editors of several leading biomedical journals have similar worries, and they recently forged a common editorial policy that was adopted and subsequently published simultaneously in several journals.[4] Concerned with the commercialization of research, they wished to protect their journals from being a 'party to potential misrepresentation.' The editors especially oppose contract research, where participating researchers often do not have access to the full range of data that play a role in the final version of the submitted article. The new guidelines are part of a revised document known as 'Uniform Requirements for Manuscripts Submitted to Biomedical Journals,'[5] a compendium of guidelines used by many leading biomedical journals. Here, in outline, are the relevant main points:

- Authors must disclose any financial relations they have that might bias their work. For example: are they shareholders in the company that funded the study or manufactures the product? Are they paid consultants? At the journal editor's discretion, this information would be published along with the report.
- Researchers should not enter into agreements that restrict in any way their access to the full data, nor should they be restricted in contributing to the interpretation and analysis of that data.
- Journal editors and reviewers should similarly avoid conflicts of interest in the peer review process.

These guidelines, if rigorously enforced, should go a long way in helping improve the situation. In fact, I think the journals have come close to doing everything they can do.[6] But it still is not enough.

Notice how little journal policy will matter when it comes to self-censorship. The new regulations that I mentioned above will – at best – ensure that any work that does get done meets a certain threshold of scientific legitimacy. But the problem with self-censorship is that some types of work will not be done at all, or, if done, will not be reported. And there is nothing that any journal can do about that. I will come back to this point below.

Stunningly, one journal reversed its adoption of a related policy. The *New England Journal of Medicine* has modified the part of its policy applicable to review articles that survey and evaluate various commercial products, which previously said, 'authors of such articles will not have any financial interest in a company (or its competitor) that makes a product discussed in the article.' The new policy says: 'authors of such articles will not have any *significant* financial interest in a company (or its competitor) that makes a product discussed in the article' (my italics).[7] The addition of 'significant' makes quite a difference. Anything up to $10,000 is considered acceptable. The reasons for this policy change are particularly worrisome. The journal editors think that concerns about bias should not arise until significant sums are involved. Perhaps they are right. But it should be noted that someone with 'insignificant' commercial connections to several different companies could be adding $50,000 to $100,000 to her income without violating the new journal rules.

The editors also claim in their editorial – and this is shocking – that it is increasingly difficult to find people to do reviews who do not have economic ties to the corporate world.[8] If they omitted such reviews, they would publish nothing at all on new products, leaving readers with no means of evaluation except that provided by the manufacturers themselves. Jeffrey Drazen remarked that he was able to commission only one review in the two years he has edited the journal. The suggestion is that moderately biased information is better than no information. If it is true that almost all reviewers have corporate ties – and I shudder to think it may be so – then the current situation is even worse than any reasonable paranoid would have feared.

Critics of commercialized research tend to focus on moral improprieties, such as a lack of informed consent. My concerns are entirely epistemic. That is, I am worried about the quality of the scientific knowledge, not the mistreatment of people in acquiring it. Many of these problems, both moral and epistemic, can be controlled, at least in principle, by regulation. Conflict of interest rules should be able to prevent abuses of the sort I mentioned, though not without difficulty. Finder's fees, for example, are sometimes paid to physicians who enrol patients in clinical trials. The existence of such fees is a major source of concern, since inappropriate subjects are being recruited. But the finder's fee can be hidden in so-called administrative costs, thus concealing the otherwise evident conflict. In any case, most discussion of these issues focuses on regulating conflict of interest,[9] whereas there is an epistemic problem independent of these considerations, which cannot be controlled by the same sorts of conflict of interest regulations. The problems described so far are sins of commission. The problems I have in mind are more like sins of omission and they stem from various forms of self-censorship.

The epistemic problem is a lack of alternative theories, and it is to this type of problem that I now wish to turn. The point is so obvious, and so important, that it hardly needs mentioning, yet it is often overlooked. Corporations understandably want a return on their investments. The pay-off for research comes from the royalties generated by patents. This means corporations will tend only to fund things that could in principle result in a patent. Other kinds of information are financially useless and might even prove financially harmful.

Imagine two ways of approaching a health problem: one involves the development of a new drug, the other focuses on, say, diet and exercise. The second could well be a far superior treatment, both cheaper and more beneficial. But it will not be funded by corporate sponsors, since there is not a penny to be made from the unpatentable research results. A source of funding that does not have a stake in the outcome, but simply wants to know how best to treat a human ailment, in contrast, would happily fund both approaches in order to determine which is superior. Public funding is clearly the answer to this problem.

Even within patentable research, some areas will be less profitable than others. Diseases of the poor and the Third World (e.g., malaria) thus remain relatively unexplored, since the poor cannot afford to pay high royalties. Hence, we find another form of self-censorship: privately funded researchers choose to ignore certain medical problems, however scientifically interesting and socially important, because they are financially unrewarding.

We are also in danger of losing a genuine resource in the form of top-notch researchers who do not do patentable work because of the nature of the discipline. Berkeley once had a Division of Biological Control and a Department of Plant Pathology, but neither exist today.[10] Why? Some people close to the scene speculate that it is simply because the type of work done in these units is not profitable. Typical research involved the study of natural organisms in their environments carried out with a view to controlling other natural organisms. This type of work cannot be patented. Is it profitable? No. Is it valuable? Yes.

Trends being the way they are, top graduate students will not go into that field. Fewer and fewer people will work on agricultural and environmental problems through biological control. Perhaps the petrochemical industry will be able to solve all our agricultural problems. It is not the job of a philosopher to speculate on this possibility. But it is the job of the philosophy of science to point out that without seriously funded rival approaches, we will never know how good or bad particular patentable solutions really are. So we have yet another form of harmful self-censorship, this time in the choice of area of research when entering graduate school.

The epistemic point is a commonplace among philosophers. Evaluation is a comparative process, and the different background assumptions of rival theories lead us to see the world in different ways. Rival research programs can be compared in terms of their relative success over the long run, but comparison requires strong rivals. It is hard to overemphasize this point. I hope I can be forgiven for making a dogmatic assertion about the nature of research in general. Scientific theories are not simply tested by comparing them with nature; they are tested and evaluated comparatively. Crucially important features of any theory or method of medical treatment are revealed only by contrast with rival theories and rival techniques. A theory that lacks a spectrum of rivals is no better tested and evaluated than a boxer who has never been in the ring with another prizefighter.[11]

This leads us to another form of self-censorship: deliberate ignorance. There is some reason to believe that the tobacco industry took legal advice to the effect that they should not do any research into the possible harmful effects of tobacco.[12] Had they come to know of any harmful effects, this would have greatly increased their legal liability. When such information came into their hands, they naturally tried to suppress it, but from their viewpoint, it is better not to know about it in the first place. Given the potential lawsuits over liability, ignorance is bliss. Interestingly, many of the lawyers who advise the tobacco industry also advise pharmaceutical companies. The legal firm of Shook, Hardy and Bacon, for instance, advises both the tobacco industry and Eli Lilly.[13]

This legal strategy assumes a distinction philosophers know well – the distinction between discovery and justification. The thinking seems to be that vague suggestions that tobacco causes lung cancer, or that Selective Serotonin Reuptake Inhibitors (SSRIs), sometimes induce suicide are just that – vague. They are mere hunches based on limited study and anecdotal reports. These reports, it is claimed, do not constitute evidence; real evidence would require extensive clinical trials. Since these trials have not been done, we have no evidence at all. There is no justification, according to the relevant companies, for making claims about the harmfulness of tobacco or SSRIs.

There is a great deal of naivety about so-called scientific method, sometimes amounting to wilful ignorance. Some researchers claim that clinical trials are both necessary and sufficient for definite knowledge, and anything short of a full clinical trial is useless. This all-or-nothing attitude is ridiculous. We choose which clinical trials to run on the basis of plausibility; circumstantial and anecdotal considerations play a role in choosing which theory to develop and test. This, too, is evidence, though usually not as strong. Often, these plausibility considerations are enough – or should be enough – to launch a serious study.

Refusing to take action on the grounds that there is nothing but 'anecdotal evidence' is atrociously bad philosophy of science, and as a form of self-censorship it can have criminal consequences. Even the Nazis established the link between smoking and lung cancer in the 1930s.[14] Commercial interests elsewhere stood in the way for decades, during which time millions of people died.

I mentioned SSRIs, which are widely used in combatting depression. Prozac is perhaps the best known of these drugs. There is a lot of interesting stuff to be discovered here. In some cases, SSRIs may actually improve extremely depressed people's condition to the point where they are capable of suicide. This sounds paradoxical, but what seems to happen in those cases is that extremely depressed people are sometimes in a 'non-responsive or lethargic' state and the SSRI will improve their condition to the point where they have the energy and the wherewithal to commit suicide. At the other end of the spectrum, even some healthy, non-depressed volunteers have become suicidal after taking SSRIs. Needless to say, this is something a profit-seeking corporation is reluctant to investigate.

David Healy, a British psychiatrist currently serving as director of the North Wales Department of Psychological Medicine at the University of Wales, has spoken and written extensively on mental illness, especially on pharmaceuticals and their history.[15] In September 2000, he was offered and accepted a position as director of the Mood and Anxiety Disorders Program in the Centre for Addiction and Mental Health (CAMH), which is affiliated with the University of Toronto. As part of the deal, he was also appointed professor in the university's Department of Psychiatry. Before he moved permanently to Canada Healy took part in a Toronto conference in November 2000, and gave a talk that was quite critical of the pharmaceutical industry. Among other things, he claimed that Prozac and other SSRIs can cause suicides. Within days of this talk, CAMH withdrew the appointment. Healy was, in effect, fired before he started. Needless to say, this caused quite a scandal. CAMH claims that they realized they had made a mistake, that Healy would not be a suitable appointment on purely academic grounds. Others suggest that pressure from Eli Lilly did him in. I doubt both of these explanations. Much more plausible is the view that self-censorship was at play. Lilly contributes financially to CAMH, a fact that lends some credence to this speculation. In such an atmosphere, self-censorship works very effectively.

We need not worry about the details of the Healy case; the crucial point is that it is not in Eli Lilly's interest to 'know' that Prozac causes suicide, since that would increase their potential liability. One might be forgiven for wondering if Eli Lilly censors itself so as to maintain a favourable legal position and CAMH censors itself so as to maintain an important source of funding. It is a case of symbiotic ignorance. The result is that an important line of research is not pursued. If work is to be done on this issue, it will have to be publicly funded: Lilly is unlikely to foot the bill.

This brings me back to the journals. The only research that will be scrutinized for conflict of interest is *submitted* research. No one makes any declarations about unsubmitted work. Imagine the following scenario. Corporation X has been making and selling product Y, but now wants to expand the medical uses for Y and so sponsors research at several universities and hospitals. Participating researchers pass on their data to corporation X, who analyse it and discover that Y is detrimental to people's health. They stop the study and submit nothing for publication. No participating scientist has access to the full data, but since nothing is submitted to any journal, no one is required by journal policy to have access to it. The dangers of Y go unreported. This scenario is completely compatible with the journal requirement that researchers have access to all the data. The sponsor willingly complies in full – nothing will be submitted for publication without everyone seeing all the data. This important principle is not violated so long as nothing is submitted. Obviously, we have a huge problem with yet another form of self-censorship, a problem nicely illustrated by the Olivieri case.

Nancy Olivieri is a haematologist working at a research hospital affiliated with the University of Toronto. She was working under contract on a project for Apotex, a major Canadian pharmaceutical company. She discovered (or at least believed that she discovered) that a certain drug, deferiprone, in common use and manufactured by Apotex, had some rather harmful side effects hitherto unknown. It turns out that her contract with Apotex forbade disclosure of her results without Apotex's permission. She published anyway, in spite of being warned not to do so, and was dismissed from her position. Subsequently, there was a public uproar, the University of Toronto intervened (largely because of the public scandal and the actions of the Faculty Association), and she was reinstated. Some new guidelines for corporate-sponsored work have been drawn up, but several issues in the Olivieri case remain unresolved.[16]

Once the details of the case are described, the moral for epistemology is trivial and obvious. When relevant information is withheld, the quality of our scientific beliefs is not as good as it could be. Private, profit-seeking funding for research interferes with good science.

There is clearly nothing any biomedical journal can do about this. We might imagine insisting that any research started must be completed and reported, but enforcing such a policy could be a bureaucratic nightmare. There are often very good reasons to stop in the middle of a project, reasons that have nothing to do with wanting to hide the facts. The experiment might, for example, be found to be poorly designed, while with suitable modifications a much better one could be started. Doubtless there is more to be said on this point.

Perhaps the participating scientists would suspect that something is amiss and demand to know why the study was being stopped. But this is to expect too much of ordinary, decent people who are unlikely to risk their careers and future funding opportunities on the basis of a hunch. Olivieri has been put through the wringer, and even received anonymous letters disparaging her and her supporters.[17] Others censor themselves in these sorts of situations. They will not lie when asked by a journal editor to sign a form explicitly declaring their financial connection to corporation X, but they are not likely to go out of their way to make trouble for themselves. Peter Desbarats, a former dean of journalism at the University of Western Ontario, commented on his own self-censorship in a similar type of situation:

> The moment of truth arrived for me in 1995, when Rogers Communications granted my request for $1 million to endow a chair of information studies, for which I was extremely grateful. When journalists subsequently asked me to comment on the subsequent Rogers takeover of Maclean Hunter, all I could do was draw their attention to the donation. They understood right away that I had been, to express it crudely, bought.
>
> This had nothing to do with Rogers. I had begged for the money. It was given with no strings attached. It will serve a useful purpose. But unavoidably, I gave up something in return. No one should ever pretend, least of all university presidents, that this experience, multiplied many times and repeated over the years, doesn't damage universities in the long run.[18]

Let me quickly head off an objection I have heard more than once: if Apotex had not provided the funds for Olivieri's research in the first place, there would have been no discovery about the harmful side effects. Since they are not morally or legally obliged to fund research, they should not be morally or legally obliged to make the results known when they do fund it. The problem with this reply is twofold. First, I am not obliged to go for a walk in the woods, but if I do and come across someone in desperate need (a hiker with a broken leg, for example), then I am certainly obliged to help. Second, and this is by far the more important point, we should not be thinking in terms of private funding for research versus no funding. The real dichotomy is private versus public funding. The alternative to Apotex paying the research bills is to have public money provide the support. A public funder would not have any financial interest in suppressing results.

Broadly speaking, I see four ways of dealing with the problem of the commercialization of research and the self-censorship that attends it: (1) deny or ignore it; (2) just live with it; (3) introduce regulations to cope with it; or (4) introduce full public funding and eliminate commercial interests for all medical research. The first two suggestions do not merit comment; the latter two should be taken seriously.

The regulation route has much to recommend it. Many of the problems with the commercialization of research can be mitigated by carefully constructed rules that are rigorously enforced. The biomedical journal policy that I described above, for instance, will go a long way towards catching and preventing many of the more blatant abuses that have arisen. In responding to the Olivieri case, Ferris, Singer, and Naylor[19] also take the view that better governance will solve the problems. Unfortunately, they rather naively think there will be no problems with private funding for research as long as it is properly regulated. But there are problems that such regulations cannot solve. I mentioned one such problem above, with respect to the new journal policy requiring financial disclosure and full availability of all data to the researchers involved. I will reiterate it now. While the new regulations will ensure that any work that gets published meets a certain threshold of scientific legitimacy, some types of work simply will not get done, or if done, will not get reported. I stress that this is quite different from the problem of fraudulent reporting. Regulation might be able to control fraud, but there is nothing that any journal or regulatory body can do about self-censorship. They cannot oversee or referee work that is not done or is not submitted, whatever the reason.[20]

I have been hinting throughout this paper at the solution to these very serious problems – a return to public funding and public control

of all medical research. Given the size and influence of private involvement in research, calling for an exclusively public science may seem a
radical step. Perhaps it is, but there is an obvious analogy that makes it
seem a little less extreme. Socialized medicine is unquestionably better
than its market-driven alternative – it is universal, it is cheaper, and so
on. Even though it would be a very radical change for some countries
(the United States in particular) to switch to socialized medicine, most
knowledgeable people (who are not in a conflict of interest position
because of a financial relation to the private medical or insurance
industries) think that the overhaul would be a very good thing. In calling for the socialization of medical research, I am calling for something
less radical than the introduction of socialized medicine *de novo*.
Rather, we should view it as a modest extension of the existing system
of socialized medicine.

Even less ambitiously, we could simply call for a return to the funding systems that were in place twenty-five years ago, before the *Bayh-
Dole Act* of 1980. The then reigning spirit was captured in a 1948 declaration by Yale University: 'It is, in general, undesirable and contrary to
the best interests of medicine and the public to patent any discovery or
invention applicable in the fields of public health or medicine.'[21] I have
a preference for something more systematic than the old system of
support, so let me suggest some avenues that should be further
explored.

I see socialized research consisting in the following. First, government funding would be provided for all important medical research.
This would be conducted at universities and also, perhaps, at dedicated institutions. The level of support would be a political decision, of
course, but it should cover both the existing public funding for
research and a substantial part of what private industry currently
invests in research. It need not match, since much private research
money is for research related to marketing, and for the pursuit of
so-called me too drugs that merely replicate existing profitable drugs
produced by a rival company. Neither of these expenses is in any way
beneficial or necessary. The abolition of patents, or fundamental
changes to the patent system, should also be considered, so that industry patents do not hinder publicly funded research

These suggestions need, of course, to be further developed by people with appropriate expertise in drug policy, regulation, and econom-
ics. Public policy is highly complex and requires a level of expertise
that I do not have. Nevertheless, a proposal along these lines is one

way to solve the spectrum of problems associated with privately funded research and its attendant self-censorship. Like ordinary censorship, self-censorship is the enemy of good science. It is a terrible betrayal in any branch of knowledge; in medical research it is wantonly criminal.

NOTES

1 R.A. Davidson, 'Sources of Funding and Outcome of Clinical Trials' (1986) 12 J. Gen. Intern. Med. 155.
2 Mark Friedberg et al., 'Evaluation of Conflict of Interest in New Drugs Used in Oncology' (1999) 282 J. Am. Med. Assoc. 1453.
3 Henry Thomas Stelfox et al., 'Conflict of Interest in the Debate over Calcium-Channel Antagonists' (1998) 338 New Eng. J. Med. 101.
4 For instance, Frank Davidoff, 'Sponsorship, Authorship, and Accountability' (2001) 358 Lancet 854. It can also be found in the mid-September issues of 2001 of the *New England Journal of Medicine*, the *Journal of the American Medical Association*, and others.
5 International Committee of Medical Journal Editors, 'Uniform Requirements for Manuscripts Submitted to Biomedical Journals: Writing and Editing for Biomedical Publication.' http://www.icmje.org/index.html.
6 One thing they still might do is insist that every clinical trial be registered at the outset. No results would be accepted for publication unless they were registered. Thus, if negative results are discovered but not published, others can raise questions. Conversation between Catherine DeAngelis, the editor of the *Journal of American Medical Association*, and the author.
A proposal along these lines has just been adopted by leading medical journals. For a brief report see www.newscientist.com/news/news.jsp?id =ns999963. This very welcome development has some effect on claims made in this paper, but not on the central point that regulation cannot cure all the ills of the commercialization of medical research, or even most of the important ones associated with self-censorship.
7 Jeffrey M. Drazen and Gregory D. Curfman, 'Editorial' (2002) 346 New Eng. J. Med. 1901 [emphasis added].
8 It should be noted that Jerome Kassirer, the preceding editor of the *New England Journal of Medicine*, sharply disagreed; see John McKenzie, 'Conflict of Interest? Medical Journal Changes Policy of Finding Independent Doctors to Write' (12 June 2002), http://www.vaccinationnews.com/dailynews/june2002/conflictofinter est14.htm.

9 For instance, Trudo Lemmens and Paul B. Miller, 'The Human Subjects Trade: Ethical and Legal Issues Surrounding Recruitment Incentives' (2003) 31 J.L. Med. & Ethics 398, explore the use of various regulatory and legal sanctions, including those based on criminal law, to deal with conflict of interest.

10 Eyal Press and Jennifer Washburn, 'The Kept University' Atlantic (March 2000), http://www.theatlantic.com/issues/2000/03/press.htm.

11 For more on this point and on so-called scientific method in general, see James Robert Brown, Who Rules in Science: An Opinionated Guide to the Wars (Cambridge, MA: Harvard University Press, 2001).

12 Seth Shulman, Owning the Future (New York: Houghton Mifflin, 1999).

13 Ibid.

14 Robert N. Proctor, The Nazi War on Cancer (Princeton, NJ: Princeton University Press, 1999).

15 See David Healy, The Creation of Psychopharmacology (Cambridge, MA: Harvard University Press, 2001).

16 See Jon Thompson, Patricia Baird, and Jocelyn Downie, 'Report of the Committee of Inquiry on the Case Involving Dr. Nancy Olivieri, the Hospital for Sick Children, the University of Toronto, and Apotex, Inc.,' http://www.caut.ca/english/issues/acadfreedom/olivieri.asp.

17 Ibid. at 9, 383 et seq.

18 Peter Desbarats, 'Who's on the Barricades?' Globe and Mail, 3 June 1998, A21.

19 Lorraine E. Ferris, Peter A. Singer, and C. David Naylor, 'Better Governance in Academic Health Sciences Centres: Moving Beyond the Olivieri/Apotex Affair in Toronto' (2004) 30 J. Med. Ethics 25.

20 Between the time of the first version of the paper and the one that is going to press, a number of medical journals adopted a policy of requiring the registration of clinical trials. This is a very important new regulation and will address some (but certainly not all) of my concerns. See Catherine D. DeAngelis, et al., 'Clinical Trial Registration' (2004) 292 J. Am Med. Assoc. 1363, http://jama.ama-assn.org/cgi/content/full/292/11/1363.

21 Archie M. Palmer, Survey of University Patent Policies: Preliminary Report (Washington, DC: National Research Council, 1948) at 76.

6 Promoting Integrity in Industry-Sponsored Clinical Drug Trials: Conflict of Interest Issues for Canadian Health Sciences Centres

LORRAINE E. FERRIS AND C. DAVID NAYLOR

Canadians have an interest in gaining access to safe and efficacious new drugs, while manufacturers have a related interest in developing pharmaceutical agents and moving them to market. The process of regulatory approval for new drugs seeks to align these interests through safeguards to prevent introduction of drugs that are inefficacious for their stated indications, or that have unacceptable risk-benefit ratios owing to serious adverse effects.

Investigational drugs typically first undergo animal toxicity and pharmacokinetic studies. A sponsor (e.g., the pharmaceutical manufacturer)[1] can then apply to Health Canada's Therapeutic Products Directorate (TPD) for entry into the pre-approval process. This authorizes the manufacturer to begin controlled clinical trials of the agent with human subjects. Ideally, scientifically rigorous methods are used to compare outcomes between the new agent and usual treatments for a particular clinical condition. These methods are designed to enhance the accuracy and precision of the evidence arising from studies of particular drugs.

Sponsors can only undertake these studies by interacting with clinicians and facilities or institutions that provide care for the patient populations in whom the drugs can be tested. These interactions may be direct, or mediated through contract research organizations of one type or another.

All involved ideally should share the goal of designing, conducting, and reporting these clinical trials with scientific integrity. However, the sponsor will almost invariably have invested a substantial amount of time and money in the pre-clinical and pre-approval stages of drug development. Delays or negative outcomes of trials can have adverse financial consequences for sponsors.[2] As well, the infusion of corporate funding of clinical trial research into the health sector creates potential conflicts of interest (COIs) for the investigators and facilities who benefit financially and in other ways from their interactions with industry.

As any sponsorship of clinical research by an investor-owned third party can be seen as creating apparent COI, there is some attraction in separating actual COI from other types of COI. One observer has suggested the adoption of less accusatory terminology, the 'appearance of a partiality problem,'[3] when referring to potential or apparent conflict of interest. In this paper we stay with the term COI for actual, apparent, and potential situations, with the caveat that COIs are ubiquitous and vary in their seriousness. Following Thompson, we define a COI as a 'set of conditions in which professional judgment concerning a primary interest (e.g., a patient's welfare or the validity of research) tends to be unduly influenced by a secondary interest (e.g., financial gain).'[4]

These COIs may be financial or non-financial, and operate at either the individual (physician or clinical investigator) or institutional (site) level.[5] Individual COIs mostly occur when physicians acting as clinical investigators are financially rewarded (e.g., monetarily, or via gifts, bonuses, stock options, or equipment) for their involvement in the clinical trial. The financial mechanisms include finders' fees for referring, identifying, and/or recruiting research subjects, and completion fees for having successfully retained a research subject in a trial. Other rewards may include over-compensation for services rendered, or compensation for usual care when these services are already the subject of a third-party reimbursement scheme or other cost-recovery mechanisms. Individuals may also be paid for trial involvement by the provision of general consulting arrangements. Non-financial conflicts of interest include authorship of publications reporting on the trial results in peer-reviewed journals, peer and institutional recognition, and career advancement.

Institutional COI mostly occurs when the Academic Health Sciences Centre (AHSC) or non-AHSC hospital accepts financial rewards for administering a trial (e.g., inflated overhead charges) or other compensation for participating in a trial (e.g., donations for research or other university or hospital programs). Either the institution or the clinical investigator may also hold some or all of the commercial rights to the pharmaceutical agent, creating a particularly direct COI as regards the results of the trial. Institutions have non-financial COI analogous to those for the individuals working on site.

Canada's publicly funded health care system in itself does not provide any particular protections against these COI. On the contrary, because professional fees and institutional funding envelopes are capped, revenues from industry-sponsored trials are doubly attractive. These revenues are also defended as promoting the public good since they provide financing for other hospital research programs or clinical services.

As already noted, actual, potential, or apparent COI is more or less ubiquitous in the context of industry-sponsored clinical studies. There are accordingly two ways forward. One, more post hoc than preventive, is to study each set of circumstances[6] and determine whether a reasonable observer would be concerned about the COI inherent in the research. The second is to devise and implement policies that prevent or mitigate COI, or that facilitate the identification of relevant COI on the part of those involved in designing, conducting, and reporting industry-sponsored drug studies.

Against this background, we examine how AHSCs can promote integrity in industry-sponsored clinical drug trials that offer the foundational evidence on which regulatory drug approval rests. We refer to these studies as 'pre-approval clinical drug trials.' We set aside evaluation of medical devices, given their separate regulatory machinery, but readers should be aware that there are overlapping issues.[7] Although we focus on Canadian AHSCs, selected comparisons with the United States are drawn for illustrative purposes. Canadian AHSCs do differ from each other in structure, size, and research culture; however, the issues raised in this chapter should be broadly applicable to Canadian AHSCs.

Definitions used in this chapter are provided in the appendix, while table 6.1 reviews various types of COI for ease of reference. The remainder of the chapter is divided into three parts. Part I elaborates on (a) issues concerning conflicts of interest; (b) the context in which pre-approval clinical trials are conducted in Canada; (c) the pharmaceutical industry in Canada; (d) the Canadian system for regulating drugs; and (e) features of an academic health sciences complex. Part II reviews some of the relevant literature on integrity of industry-sponsored clinical trials, with particular reference to financial COI in AHSCs. Part III offers some recommendations for mechanisms to promote the integrity of industry-sponsored research in the Canadian context.

I. Context for Industry-Sponsored Clinical Trials in Canada

COI and Industry-Sponsored Clinical Trials

The harms from COI in clinical trials fall into two broad categories: harm to the actual research subjects, and harms to other patients and the broad public interest when invalid research results mislead regulators and result in suboptimal clinical practices.

David Blumenthal has pointed out that while there is no definitive evidence that COI has directly injured a research subject, a number of cases have 'certainly created the suspicion or appearance of that eventuality.'[8] For example, as discussed in previous chapters, Jesse Gelsinger died in a clinical trial testing a gene transfer vector developed at the Institute for Human Gene Therapy, a division of the University of Pennsylvania. The institute had commercial rights to the treatment, and the physician investigators were university hospital medical staff. Along with the university, they held equity positions in the company that owned the commercial rights of the research and they administered the vector. These financial interests, as well as others disclosed in the plaintiff's lawsuit, were not revealed to potential research subjects.[9] Other lawsuits by families of research subjects have likewise raised concerns about COI in industry-sponsored research.[10]

Such concerns are not new. A U.S. congressional committee hearing in 1989 brought the question of COI in industry-sponsored clinical studies forcibly to public attention.[11] One case considered in the hearing involved very favourable initial reports on Tretinoin based on research by a Harvard academic. The company went public and its stock rose significantly after the report. The researcher did not disclose his involvement in forming the company that manufactured Tretinoin, or that he owned stock. After the researcher cashed in his shares, the manufacturer announced that the earlier positive results from the clinical trials were premature and the stock fell. The researcher was accused of holding back negative clinical trial results until after he had secured his financial interests.

Another case concerned the NIH-funded multi-site TIMI trials that compared the effectiveness of two thrombolytic agents (t-PA and streptokinase) for treating heart attacks. The first findings showed statistically significant differences between the two agents in favour of t-PA. Five of the authors had stock in the company that manufactured t-PA, and the reporting of favourable results led to a rise in the stock price. None of the researchers declared their equity interests in the pharmaceutical company. Other groups without stock interests found the two agents relatively comparable. The Committee on Conflicts of Interest said, 'the research literature on t-PA has repeated examples of more positive evaluations of t-PA by scientists with relationships with Genentech, compared to scientists without such relationships.'[12] Since NIH at that time lacked a COI policy, they were unaware of the stock ownership. The congressional hearings led to regulatory changes in NIH and eventually to changes to the U.S. Food and Drug Administration (FDA). Intriguingly, the TIMI observations have been validated by various investigators, but the controversy about the respective merits of t-PA and streptokinase has continued for more than a decade.

The chronicle continues with respect to t-PA, albeit for another indication: stroke, rather than heart attack. In 2002, the *British Medical Journal* published a report[13] stating that the majority of the American Heart Association's experts for a five-year multi-site trial on t-PA for stroke (1995)[14] had ties to the drug's manufacturer. The FDA approved t-PA for the treatment of acute ischemic stroke in June 1996. Again, however, there are many experts who believe that t-PA is actually underused for acute stroke and represents the only effective treatment on the market today.

The situation with t-PA illustrates the knife edge on which management of COI must balance. It is not in the public interest to unreasonably reduce the number and kinds of sites involved in clinical trials or to prohibit the involvement of experienced clinical investigators in industry-sponsored research. Interpreting trial data can be difficult at the best of times, and reasonable people will disagree, sometimes heatedly, about evidence from clinical trials. Apparent or actual COI in the design, conduct, and reporting of trials adds layers of uncertainty that make the interpretation of trial evidence even more challenging. Allowing seriously flawed overestimation of the probability of risk or implausible associations to dominate discourse about public issues is, as Alvin Weinberg says, 'hardly less fatuous than were the witch-hunts of the Middle Ages.'[15] Indeed, a form of non-financial COI can be perceived as regards the conduct of moral entrepreneurs in the bioethics and clinical research communities whose careers may be advanced by their self-proclaimed 'watch-dog' or 'whistle-blowing' activities regarding the influence of industry in clinical research. The challenge is to prevent, detect, and control the influence of COI in an effective, transparent, and equitable fashion.

Canadian Pre-Approval Clinical Trial Research

In Canada, the usual model for pre-approval clinical drug trials involves a contractual relationship ('clinical trial agreement') between a private pharmaceutical company ('sponsor'), a physician ('qualified investigator'), and the clinical site ('site'). These clinical trials are regulated by federal legislation under the authority of Health Canada. In some cases, clinical investigators may organize themselves into networks that work directly with industry, but such networks are unusual and will not be addressed directly in this chapter.

In the United States, federal agencies do fund clinical trials that are integral to FDA approval under a 'bench to bedside' mandate.[16] This mandate is less developed in Canada. The Canadian Institutes of Health Research (CIHR) do not provide the sole source of funding for pre-approval clinical trials of drugs, opting instead to fund pre-clinical biomedical research and clinical trials in areas that would be less interesting to industry.

The legislative landscape is also different between Canada and the United States. There are long-standing legislative incentives (e.g., the *Bayh-Dole Act* and the *Stevenson-Wydler Technology Innovations Act*)[17] to increase collaboration between American universities (their departments and their researchers) and industry by allowing for intellectual property from federally funded research to be transferred to those who conducted the research.[18] Canada does not have analogous legislation. In the United States, when federal funds are given, the involved agency (usually the NIH) maintains and enforces policies that obligate clinical sites and clinical investigators to report on their COI. Again, Canada has not moved forward on this front, a point we revisit below.

The Pharmaceutical Industry in Canada

The pharmaceutical industry in Canada is growing. According to Industry Canada, there were 118 active pharmaceutical and medicine manufacturing sites in 1992 compared to 257 in 2001, with an accompanying rise in net revenue from $2.3 billion to 3.6 billion.[19] In 2001 the Patented Medicine Prices Review Board[20] reported that total Canadian sales by all manufacturers of pharmaceuticals for humans had risen an average of 10 per cent each year since 1998 and were estimated at $13.1 billion in 2002.[21] Canadian pharmaceutical sales account for only 2.6 per cent of the major world markets (by comparison, the United States accounts for 53.4 per cent). However, sales in Canada have grown faster in recent years than in other major markets, including that of the United States.[22]

Canada is trying to attract research and development activities in the pharmaceutical field. Industry Canada has written that '[t]he generous fiscal incentives, along with an extensive network of research-intensive hospitals, universities and government laboratories, make Canada an ideal place to conduct research and development and establish strategic partnerships. Canada also has a significant contract research industry, with many firms highly regarded internationally for their ability to conduct clinical trials.'[23] As well, the comparative costs of doing clinical research are much lower in Canada than the United States,[24] and the universal health insurance system means that a broader cross-section of patients passes through any participating clinical site.

Whatever its reasons, industry has taken a growing interest in Canada as a site for pre-approval clinical drug trials. In 2002, Canada had 1,287 new clinical trial applications[25] and 692 amendments to past clinical trial applications.[26] That same year, Health Canada approved twenty-six new active substances from fourteen different pharmaceutical companies.[27]

The Canadian System for Regulating Drugs or Medical Devices

Originally enacted in 1953 and periodically amended since by Parliament, Canada's *Food and Drugs Act*[28] governs the regulation of drugs, medical devices, other therapeutic products, food, and cosmetics.[29] The act mandates that drugs (prescription and over the counter), medical devices and other therapeutic products be tested for their safety, efficacy and quality. These regulations[30] are made under the act and unlike its parent statute, may be amended by the governor-general-in council.

The Therapeutic Products Directorate (TPD) of Health Canada has the federal authority to regulate pharmaceutical drugs and medical devices for human use.[31] The authorization to sell or import a drug used for the purposes of a clinical trial is issued to an eligible sponsor,[32] who must conduct the trials in accordance with the Good Clinical

Practice Guideline (GCP)[33] among other guidelines. Prior to being given market authorization, the act requires a sponsor to produce rigorous evidence about the quality, efficacy, and safety of investigational drugs. As noted earlier, any sponsor of an investigational drug or device can apply to the TPD to undergo the approval process after preclinical testing of the new drug in animals.[34]

The first time an investigational drug or device is given to humans is in Phase I studies. These studies are small, conducted to determine the safety and pharmacology of the new drug, and usually involve healthy subjects. Phase II clinical trials examine the short-term pharmacological properties of the compound and collect uncontrolled and preliminary information about the drug's efficacy.[35] Usually these studies are larger than those in Phase I but involve no more than several hundred people. Phase II clinical trials use patients with specific diseases or conditions. Phase III clinical trials are designed to determine the efficacy of the investigational drug and its short-term toxicities. These trials are typically large, involving anywhere from several hundred to thousands of people who have a specific disease or condition for which the drug or device could be prescribed, if it were available on the market. Phase III trials collect evidence about outcomes of direct relevance such as survival, functional status, markers of disease activity, and quality of life. Clinical trials (especially Phase II and III trials) are often multi-site, since there is a need for a large and diverse patient population. If the sponsor is seeking to have the investigational drug approved in more than one country, there may be parallel clinical trials in several countries.

The Canadian regulations recognize the importance of research ethics boards (REBs) in protecting research subjects. An REB unaffiliated with the sponsor must approve the initiation and conduct periodic review of the research to protect the rights, safety, and well-being of clinical trial subjects. Furthermore, the REB must be constituted in keeping with these regulations.[36] In Canada, however, we do not currently have federal legislation to regulate REBs. This poses problems for clinical trial research.[37] Michael McDonald has also argued that the governance of Canadian REBs is in need of major repair as regards accountability and effectiveness.[38] While accrediting and regulating REBs might address these concerns, the drawback is that REBs would become quasi-judicial bodies and act as tribunals.[39] Various Canadian groups have provided recommendations about governance models for REBs,[40] and federal legislation may be forthcoming. Enactment, however, will probably take several years,[41] and the final shape of the legislation remains unknown.

Unlike the United States, with its federal and state controls for addressing site, investigator, and REB financial COI, Canada does not have a legislative framework for COI in industry-sponsored research. For example, the United States has various controls that require investigators or sites to declare financial COI and to make available or to provide a review of the financial arrangements among the parties, while Canada's system has no such requirements.[42] Such oversight could be made consistent with the Good Clinical Practice guidelines adopted by Health Canada. Lack of explicit oversight seems ill advised, since it leaves the country without a legislative avenue to seek declarations of COI or to review the financial arrangements in a study.[43] This is not to say that the U.S. federal controls are optimal. They may not adequately reflect the complexity of COI and are not fully harmonized across the relevant government agencies. However, the U.S. controls have at least established the government's interest in providing safeguards for dealing with institutional, REB, and clinical investigator financial conflicts of interest.

In Canada, the regulations appear to rely on REBs as the mechanism to ensure that COI situations are avoided with respect to investigators and sites.[44] As we saw earlier, these boards are not directly regulated. REB members may themselves be involved in pre-approval clinical drug trials, and in these situations their colleagues are placed in the somewhat uncomfortable position of overseeing the COI of another REB member. REBs are in meaningful measure creatures of the host institution, and REB chairs, as members and staff, may be compensated by the institution or otherwise recognized for their involvement in the REB. The REB may therefore feel some obligation to facilitate conduct of revenue-generating research on site. Furthermore, the emergence of private REBs has created a problem as regards potential or actual COI in REB oversight of industry-sponsored research, notwithstanding the good intentions of those who manage and serve on these REBs. In short, the current situation leaves institutions, REBs, and investigators in an ambiguous position as regards management of COI in industry-sponsored clinical trials.

The regulations do provide for inspection of clinical trials. Under the authority of section 23 of the *Food and Drugs Act*, these inspection activities are to be conducted by the Health Products and Food Branch Inspectorate (HPFBI) and supported by the compliance and enforcement policy (POL-0001). The inspections focus on clinical trial sites (i.e., qualified investigator sites), sponsors, and contract research organizations. The main objectives for the inspection of clinical trials are to ensure that the generally accepted principles of good clinical practices are met, validate the quality of the data generated, and verify compliance to Division 5[45] of the regulations.[46]

In July 2003, the results of the first set of clinical trials inspections were issued.[47] On an annual basis, up to 2 per cent of all clinical trial sites will be inspected. For this first phase, eighteen inspections (six at sponsors' sites and twelve at qualified investigators' sites) were undertaken. The inspections focused on scientific quality of the trials and general oversight issues; they did not yield any information about COI. This is unfortunately consistent with the position of Health Canada and current legislative intent – there is neither review of financial arrangements among the parties nor review of the contractual terms and conditions. One hundred and eight deficiencies or deviations were noted; 72 per cent were from the qualified Investigators' sites. Most deficiencies in either type of site concerned records, including the maintenance of accurate clinical trial records. The second highest number of deficiencies arose from inadequate systems and procedures to ensure quality of the clinical trial. Deficiencies in informed consent constituted 14 per cent of all cases at sites of qualified investigators.

Academic Health Sciences Centres

For the most part, AHSCs are comprised of a university, its medical school, and the teaching hospitals. However, there may also be other health sciences departments, schools, or programs (e.g., nursing, pharmacy, dentistry) within an AHSC. Like other authors, we shall focus on the medical school and hospital coupling, since this is a major focus for clinical research activity within an AHSC.[48]

Any AHSC has a mixed mission comprising elements of education, research, and clinical care. Universities and their medical schools offer an academic framework for research and teaching. They supply the hospital with senior medical students and post-graduate trainees (residents) who assist with patient care. Hospitals supply clinical facilities, practical clinical experience, and access to accomplished clinical faculty who earn a livelihood within the hospital. The university and its medical school have primary responsibility for the education program; hospitals have primary responsibility for patient care issues; and both partners have responsibility for the research.[49]

A striking development in Canadian AHSCs over the past twenty years has been the emergence of major research centres within teaching hospitals and health regions. For example, at the University of Toronto, about half of all external funding flowing to investigators with faculty appointments supports work done on site at teaching hospitals. While contract research for industrial sponsors represents a rather small fraction of such funding, these are tangible sources of revenue in an environment where research dollars remain scarce. American commentators have suggested that research revenue has become a valuable means to sustain hospital missions.[50] Clinical trial research in particular can generate revenue and 'turn a hospital-based cost into a revenue source' for reinvestment into other hospital programs.[51] It has similarly been argued that revenue from clinical trials can sustain basic science laboratories and provide funding for general research purposes, including support of research fellows.[52]

It is telling that clinical trials are seen as 'profitable.' We assume the margins arise in part from the institutional overhead paid to the hospital by the sponsor, as well as the more controversial situation of payment for usual care that is already covered by hospital budgets or health insurance payments.[53] Universities presumably take a similar view of potential profit-making research endeavours, although the focus would be more likely to be on non-patient enterprises such as biotechnology more generally.

While the contributing institutions have intertwined interests and responsibilities, the nature of the relationship is dependent in part on whether the contributing institutions are affiliated with one another or whether the university owns the medical school and its teaching hospitals or vice versa.[54] In Canada, the relationship is collaborative since teaching hospitals are autonomously governed and not owned by any medical school or university. The collaboration is generally codified in an affiliation or partnership agreement.

The organizational relationships in Canadian AHSCs are further complicated by the remuneration of physicians. Physicians appointed as clinical faculty are usually classified as self-employed because their predominant source of income is payment for clinical services. Payment is most often made on a fee-per-item-of-service basis, but block payment arrangements are becoming more common across Canada. At the same time, clinical faculty often draw compensation directly from the hospital as salary (or as a stipend). Furthermore, physicians in most AHSCs have income-sharing plans, wherein clinical money pooled and reallocated to support research and educational activity. These plans are at least partly autonomous but there may be elements of co-governance with the hospital or medical school. Thus, from the standpoint of COI and industry-sponsored research, the self-employment status of physician investigators adds another layer of complexity.

Industry's business interests may conflict not only with the ethos of clinical medicine and its focus on ensuring that new drugs are indeed beneficial to patient populations, but with scholarly norms (e.g., pursuit of 'truth,' free exchange of ideas and information). Universities and their professoriate have long argued that these academic freedoms are essential for the effective discharge of the university's role as an engine of innovation and critical thinking for society. Academic freedom was first clearly articulated in 1915 by the American Association of University Professors (AAUP) in its Declaration of Principles and updated by its 1940 Statement on Principles on Academic Freedom and Tenure. Since then, interpretive comments have elaborated on the original statements and eliminated reference to countervailing responsibilities and obligations.[55]

On one level, assertions about academic freedom are part and parcel of an ideology of autonomy and non-accountability promulgated for its own purposes by occupational interest groups such as the AAUP and the Canadian Association of University Teachers. But, as is also true for professional codes of ethics, occupational ideologies are successful because they articulate values that have resonance and social utility beyond the interests of the group itself.[56] The Canadian courts, for example, have said that universities are indeed unique because they are 'self-governing centres of learning, research and teaching safeguarded by academic freedom.'[57] And the Supreme Court of Canada has described academic freedom as 'essential to our continuance as a lively democracy.'[58]

Various provisions in the CAUT definition of academic freedom are potentially at cross-purposes with the interests of industrial sponsors of clinical research, including the right to 'freedom in carrying out research and disseminating results' or 'freedom from institutional censorship.'[59] Conversely, Rebecca Eisenberg has argued that the traditional definition of academic freedom does not take into consideration issues in contract research such as how to deal with faculty members who may be in a perceived or actual COI and potentially compromise their academic values.[60] This problem, paired with institutional COI, has resulted in her claim that we need to reassess mechanisms for preserving academic freedom in sponsored research. Others have also commented on the need to protect academic freedom in contract research.[61] There have been cases where researchers have acted in good faith to conduct and report clinical research and, as a result of their research findings, have become targets of those whose financial interests were jeopardized by the research.[62]

In 2001, the Task Force on Research Accountability of the Association of American Universities published its 'Report on Individual and Institutional Financial COI.'[63] The report focuses on improving institutional mechanisms for managing COI. Implicit in this document is the view that academic freedom is owed to society and there must be mechanisms in place to prevent any university or faculty member from agreeing to limit or forfeit their academic freedom (or to be perceived to do so).

Physicians with academic appointments who work in Canadian teaching hospitals are the qualified investigators on many industry-sponsored clinical trials. The university arguably has an obligation to promote and protect the academic freedom of all faculty members, including its clinical faculty. However, there are distinct challenges in defining and protecting the academic freedom of clinical faculty. First, the academic job descriptions of many physicians vary considerably. They range from those who are primarily engaged in provision of clinical services with a limited teaching role to those who commit a major amount of time to research or education. Second, teaching hospitals have their own missions and culture; they may reasonably seek a degree of coherence, stability, and accountability that is not the norm on university campuses. Third, and as a corollary, appropriate limits must be placed on academic freedom resulting from a clinical faculty member's fiduciary obligation owed to his or her patients. In cases of doubt, the balance must fall in favour of the patient's interests. For example, academic freedom does not allow a clinical faculty member to teach outdated or harmful practices as if they were a defensible standard of practice, or to practise in an idiosyncratic fashion without reference to the norms and standards of his or her specialty.

At present, it is difficult to determine how much of the industry-sponsored clinical trial research is undertaken in Canadian AHSCs. One study estimated that between 60 and 70 per cent of protocols reviewed by Canadian research ethics boards were sponsored by industry,[64] but this does not tell us exactly where all the research was undertaken. There is some controversy about whether contract research organizations (CROs), which are private and nonacademic, are indeed competing 'head to head' with AHSCs for industry-sponsored trial business. We know that Montreal has the largest number of CROs in any North American city, suggesting that these enterprises are flourishing in some parts of Canada.[65] Certainly the International Committee of Medical Journal Editors (ICMJE) believes CROs are competing with AHSCs.[66] Thomas Bodenheimer argues that academic medical centres are less involved in clinical research than they were a decade ago because of the growth of CROs and site management organizations (SMOs).[67] His assessment is supported by figures such as a drop from 80 to 40 per cent (1991 and 1998 respectively) in the percentage of industry money going to academic medical centres and a statement in a Commonwealth Fund report that the commercial sector is able to complete clinical trials more quickly and more cheaply than AHSCs.[68] In 1998, two-thirds of all industry-sponsored clinical research projects in the United States involved a CRO.[69] CenterWatch, a clinical trials listing service, reports a recent survey showing that sponsors have dramatically increased their use of CROs for Phase II and Phase IV clinical trials and have continued to use CROs most frequently for Phase III clinical trials as well.[70] Moreover, in 2002 the rate of acquisitions within the CRO market, says CenterWatch, was five times the 2001 level, showing the monetary health of these companies. Seven of the largest global CROs agree that they have expanded the number of clinical researchers and research settings.[71] However, they argue that their research subjects are mostly drawn from primary care populations rather than from the tertiary care populations traditionally served by AHSCs. There are also examples of AHSCs transforming themselves into research networks to compete with CROs (e.g., Duke University, the University of Rochester, and the University of Pittsburgh). Canadian AHSCs have not formally adopted such strategies. However, were they to do so, additional COI concerns arise for AHSCs involved in CROs.[72]

CROs operate with a very direct financial COI: they are in the marketplace seeking business from pharmaceutical companies, and if they do not deliver positive trial outcomes, those same companies lose financially.[73] CROs usually handle the administrative aspects of a trial (including contracting with the sites and physicians and coordinating the sites for a multi-site or multi-national trial), collect data, monitor studies, and analyse data; some serve almost as an outsource option for the conduct of clinical trials. CROs often rely on independent for-profit research ethics boards, which, as noted earlier, may further compromise the integrity of the process.[74] It is uncertain whether industry in Canada is selecting CROs instead of Canadian AHSCs for clinical trials, but the concentration of CROs in Montreal suggests that this trend is accelerating here as in the United States. The American literature suggests that both community-based and academic physicians participate in CRO-managed clinical trials, but we do not know the extent to which this occurs in Canada.

II. The Integrity of Industry-Sponsored Clinical Trials

AHSCs have features that are conducive to the conduct of industry-sponsored clinical trials. First, compared to other single-site clinical settings, teaching hospitals in an AHSC have higher patient volume, more complicated cases, and more physicians who could meet the regulatory definition of a qualified investigator. While individual patients may not directly benefit from involvement in a clinical trial, such investigation offers hope for new treatments and AHSCs therefore see their role in clinical trials as important for serving the long-term public interest. There is no question that new drugs have decreased mortality and morbidity rates and improved quality of life outcomes for a variety of diseases and clinical conditions over the past fifty years.[75] However, the blurring of research integrity and corporate interests has shaken the public's trust in the clinical research enterprise and highlights the need for systemic reforms.[76]

Types and Consequences of COI

Threats to the integrity of the design, conduct, and reporting of clinical trials come from a variety of COI sources, as discussed in the introduction to this chapter and outlined in table 6.1. The various types of COI obviously overlap with each other.

The literature documents a number of concerns about the integrity of industry-sponsored trials. Among the issues identified have been the quality of clinical trials,[77] the independence of the investigators and of the AHSCs,[78] premature trial termination for financial reasons,[79] censorship or delay in publishing,[80] and low publication rates of negative trials or poorer quality of publications resulting from industry-sponsored research.[81]

Current Remedies to Deal with COI

Peer-reviewed medical journals are the gate-keepers for the dissemination of scientific discourse and research results. Journal editors have repeatedly raised and responded to concerns about the integrity of industry-sponsored clinical trials. As early as two decades ago, many peer-reviewed medical journals began requiring that authors declare their financial conflicts of interest when submitting manuscripts and stated that they may, depending upon the editorial decision, publish these with the accepted article.[82] However, a recent study found that only 43 per cent of forty-seven scientific journals responding to a questionnaire had policies requiring declaration of COI; only ten of these required disclosure of income and equity interests.[83] Another study reported that of high impact journals with policies requiring the declaration of financial conflicts of interest, only 0.05 per cent of papers included a COI declaration and 65.7 per cent published no disclosures of authors' financial COI. Medical journals were more likely than general science journals to have such disclosure requirements.[84] More generally, there appear to be differences among the types of journals with respect to what is disclosed and how disclosures are handled.[85] Journals have also addressed the growing concern that industry staff or consultants have contributed substantially to an article but are not being declared as authors.[86]

In 2001, thirteen journal editors of the ICMJE expressed concern about the influence of industry on scholarly independence and academic freedom.[87] With respect to clinical trial agreements, these editors said that they should 'give the researchers a substantial say in trial design, access to the raw data, responsibility for data analysis and interpretation, and the right to publish.'[88] For their part, editors may ask authors to state that they 'had full access to the data in the study' and 'take complete responsibility for the integrity of the data and the accuracy of the data analysis.'[89] The editors said that they would enforce adherence to the revised requirements in their 2002 uniform requirements for manuscript submission.[90] These requirements now mandate that the most responsible author sign a statement that he or she had access to the data, controlled the decision to publish, and accepts full responsibility for the conduct of the trial. The statement has been criticized for being too restrictive.[91] However, all surgical journals, among others, have since endorsed it.[92]

The *British Medical Journal* was one of the journals that did not endorse the ICMJE position, opting instead to create its own editorial policy.[93] Like the ICMJE journals, the BMJ requires disclosure of the details of all authors' and funders' roles in the study, as well as a statement that the authors accept full responsibility for the conduct of the study, had access to the data, and controlled the decision to publish. Our own view is that the ICMJE statement is too onerous and may serve to reduce the likelihood that clinical trial results are disseminated in peer-reviewed processes for critical scrutiny. The paradoxical result could be reduced transparency, as trials are submitted to regulators and used to support claims in advertisements without the usual opportunity for peer review and debate.

One large pharmaceutical company (Merck & Co., Inc.) and the Pharmaceutical Research and Manufacturers of America have issued their own statements about clinical trials that endorse different principles with weaker safeguards (the 'PhRMA principles').[94] Sponsors in general still appear to be incompletely attuned to the acuity of public and professional concerns about their role in influencing the design, conduct, and reportage of clinical research. More dialogue among AHSCs, investigators, and sponsors is needed to clarify the issues and forge greater consensus on principles, if indeed such consensus can be achieved.[95]

Among the areas for improvement and consensus is the approach to clinical trials agreements. In a study of 108 U.S. medical schools involved in industry-sponsored multi-site clinical trials research, Schulman and colleagues[96] reported that 1 per cent of agreements had clauses requiring access to trial data for authors of reports on multi-centre trials, 1 per cent required an independent data and safety monitoring board, and only 40 per cent gave full control over the publication of the study findings to investigators. These and other study results demonstrated that the ICMJE guidelines regarding trial design, data access, and publication rights were not being upheld in clinical trial agreements. We do not know if a survey of Canadian medical schools would yield similar results, but our experience suggests that the same problems occur on Canadian campuses.[97] One large Canadian academic health sciences centre has published data about the outcome of negotiations with industry regarding their AHSCs' clinical study agreements (CSAs).[98] The AHSC had agreed on three core principles governing CSAs: (1) sponsors may not suppress or otherwise censor research results; (2) investigators must retain the right to publish and to disclose immediately any safety concerns that arise during the study to their research ethics board, patients, and regulators; and (3) sponsors may require submission of research reports to them before publication to allow protection of intellectual property or debate about the interpretation of the study results, but this step is time-limited and cannot become a form of suppression. The AHSC's self-audit demonstrates that the AHSC policy was consistently implemented for managing CSAs; industrial sponsors, with few exceptions, agreed to the terms and conditions incorporated to protect academic responsibilities and public safety.[99] Unfortunately, there is still no pan-Canadian consensus on adoption of these provisions by all academic health science centres.

Various professional associations have also established guidelines and standards to address the integrity of industry-sponsored clinical trials. Many suggest that research institutions require COI disclosures and manage these by establishing various internal committees and having rules that prohibit certain activities while permitting others if these can be effectively managed. The Executive Council of the Association of American Medical Colleges (AAMC) has issued several task force reports on the issue of individual and institutional (e.g., AHSC) COI and public trust,[100] as has the Association of American Universities.[101] There are other professional guidelines and policies, such as those of the American Association of University Professors,[102] the American Medical Association, the Canadian Medical Association, and the Council of Science Editors, among others. Interestingly, some investigators in multi-centre trials have established their own stringent COI policies.[103]

AHSCs face particular challenges in dealing with COI. First, whether as self-employed professionals or as professors with the protection of academic freedom, physicians on clinical faculty will claim the right to enter into contracts and do research as they see fit. In fact, only if administrators deal with COI systematically can academic freedom be safeguarded by preventing individuals from sacrificing academic values for personal gains.[104]

Second, institutions participating in an AHSC may resist administrative regimens that interfere with their autonomy to generate revenue by striking financially favourable arrangements with pharmaceutical manufacturers.

Third, while we have highlighted some obvious instances of actual or potential COI, most situations are more subtle and may not be readily identified and recognized by the parties involved. Only with routine disclosures and systematic oversight can more subtle influences of COI be brought to light.

Fourth, the AHSC must have mechanisms in place for dealing with allegations of COI originating from within and outside the AHSC and these must be clear, capable of responding in a timely fashion, and meet the standards expected by the public. Unfortunately, AHSCs have not reached a consensus about what constitute appropriate policies and procedures for dealing with individual and institutional COI, and this has allowed institutional norms and local contexts to play a role in policy frameworks.[105] While some AHSCs have clear COI policies with oversight committees, others take a more laissez-faire approach. Peter J. Harrington has observed in his analysis of university policies that there is a difference of opinion within academia about the 'degree of danger posed by faculty conflicts of interest and the severity of restrictions that should be placed upon them.'[106] While U.S. medical schools have COI policies, these vary widely in their content and many policies are relatively weak.[107] Harvard Medical School has long been considered as having the strictest COI policy and, despite various internal reviews, has not relaxed its policy. Others have argued for similarly stringent policies to be put in place on a national basis.[108] We expect the situation with COI policies in Canada to be similar or, more likely, worse than in the United States. As noted above, in America both legislation and formal guidelines[109] have galvanized the development and implementation of policies on COI in AHSCs. No such catalyst exists in Canada.

III. Some Recommendations for Enhancing the Integrity of Industry-Sponsored Trials in Canadian AHSCs

This chapter has highlighted various threats to the integrity of industry-sponsored clinical trials arising from conflict of interest situations or the appearance of partiality. We have also reviewed some of the remedies developed and implemented to deal with COI in industry-sponsored research and noted that Canada has lagged behind the

United States regarding legislation and regulation to deal systematically with these issues. In this section, we offer some recommendations about how Canadian administrators and regulators might better prevent and manage COI in industry-sponsored clinical trials.

Local Guidelines and Policies

Various AHSCs are moving ahead with policies designed to protect the integrity of industry-sponsored clinical studies. This movement has been most visible in the Toronto academic health science complex, where there has been steady upgrading of the provisions for protecting the integrity of clinical research. However, our experience in Toronto has not been uniformly positive. There are ongoing tensions among the partners about the content and implementation of guidelines for appropriate clinical study agreements, and COI policies for the nine teaching hospitals and on-campus researchers are not harmonized. Furthermore, because the guidelines for clinical study agreements are not standardized across Canada, sponsors object to modifying contracts for Toronto sites, and there continues to be a concern that industry-sponsored clinical trials are being moved either to other AHSCs or to community hospitals and CROs. A related problem is the fact that none of the institutions have agreed on a policy for institutional COI. Sponsors can in theory skew relations with host institutions around clinical studies by offering donations or other benefits to institutions. Such COI must be publicly acknowledged by institutions, but few Canadian AHSCs or universities make any clear declaration of potential or actual institutional COI. Finally, REBs are neither consistently governed nor systematically accredited.

All of this argues for the creation of consistent policies for all AHSCs and universities. A useful first step would be for AHSCs to delineate principles they will adopt when negotiating the terms and conditions in clinical trial agreements. These principles at a minimum should ensure that investigators have the freedom to communicate directly and without censorship or inappropriate delay to the scientific community, and that they are able to meet all the current requirements of peer-reviewed journals as regards the integrity of research and their own potential or actual COIs.

However, even if such a policy could be agreed by task forces struck under the auspices of bodies such as the Association of Universities and Colleges of Canada, the Association of Canadian Medical Colleges, or the Association of Canadian Academic Healthcare Organizations, we have no guarantee that the policy would be universally adopted or consistently implemented.

COI and the Regulatory Process

We believe Canada needs to address site and investigator COI or the appearance of partiality at the time a sponsor applies to the Therapeutic Products Directorate by regulatory mechanisms. Health Canada should require mandatory declaration of COI to the TPD by investigators and sites. These declarations ought to be carefully reviewed before a sponsor is authorized to proceed. There should also be annual declarations to ensure that the situation has not significantly changed during the conduct of the trial. All such disclosure reports must be interpreted using rules clearly established in advance. To identify inappropriate inducements to investigators or sites for their participation in a trial, the relevant regulation or legislation should require a declaration of all words or conduct that involve making a promise or giving assurance to provide or accept benefits (e.g., bonuses, donations, equipment). An individual making false declarations should be regarded as having committed professional misconduct, and be reported to his or her university, the hospital, and the appropriate local self-regulatory body. In the case of institutional false declaration, we believe the reporting should be to relevant governments and granting councils.

Canada also needs to agree on a governance model for REBs and enact federal legislation to regulate them so that their work can be aligned with initiatives aimed at avoiding or containing the effects of COI. We look forward to the debate about the recommendations already made in this regard and the further debate that will accompany any draft legislation. We believe REBs should be following standardized rules for defining, determining, and managing COI. Given that clinical study agreements take legal precedence over other trial documents (e.g., policies, study protocols), we recommend that these agreements be part of the documentation that REBs review for potential COI before approving any clinical study for on-site initiation. Any rules developed to deal with COI ought to deal with matters such as how to determine reasonable compensation to investigators or sites for services or activities performed and benchmarks to be used for detecting unreasonable inducements for trial participation.[110]

Professional Self-Regulatory Bodies

We recommend that Medical Advisory Committees (MACs) and, preferably, medical regulators eliminate threats to trial integrity that are within their authority. Either through amendment of hospital by-laws or promulgation of regulations for professional conduct, MACs and medical regulators respectively should prohibit physicians from offering or accepting money or other rewards given by a sponsor (or by a physician) to a physician (or a group of physicians) in payment for identifying or recruiting a patient into a study (finders' fees), or for a patient's successful completion of the study or trial protocol (completion fees). Regulators could also have a positive effect on research practices in non-academic and non-institutional settings by publicizing the fact that it is professional misconduct for any licensed physician to undertake research without formal review by a duly constituted REB.

Mechanisms for Monitoring Site and Investigator COI

While a very important initiative and relatively new, our national inspection strategy for clinical trials is inadequate. The inspections should be wider ranging and more systematic. The inspection of research involving human subjects needs to include a review of how the research may be affected by COI. At a minimum, inspectors should assess a sample of clinical study agreements and related financial agreements to see if there are any inducements that cause legitimate concerns about the judgment of the investigators or site administration.

The GCP currently includes these study contracts as essential trial documents, thus regulatory change may not be necessary to allow for such a review. However, while review of the documents may be feasible under current regulation, regulatory amendment may be required to enable the TPD to act on the information.

Rebuilding Public Trust

Throughout this brief discussion, we have highlighted the potential and actual impacts of COI on the integrity of industry-sponsored clinical research, particularly when that research takes place in AHSCs. The evidence for subtle and not-so-subtle influences of industry on the design, conduct, analysis, and reportage of pre-approval trials of new drugs has led to growing concerns on the part of many observers about the validity of evidence used for assessing the safety and efficacy of pharmaceutical agents. While some centres in the United States and Canada have taken steps to address COI at multiple levels, we believe that the fastest way forward is through legislation and regulation that will create a more consistent platform for detecting and managing COI in industry-sponsored clinical research. Any other approach will, we fear, ultimately leave gaps in the ethical fabric for industry-sponsored drug research in Canada.

Appendix
Definitions Used in this Chapter

Conflict of interest (COI) refers to a 'set of conditions in which professional judgement concerning a primary interest (e.g., a patient's welfare or the validity of research) tends to be unduly influenced by a secondary interest (e.g., financial gain).[111]

Clinical trial means 'an investigation in respect of a drug for use in humans that involves human subjects and that is intended to discover or verify the clinical, pharmacological or pharmacodynamic effects of the drug, identify any adverse events in respect of the drug, study the absorption, distribution, metabolism and excretion of the drug or ascertain the safety or efficacy of the drug.'[112]

Clinical trial agreements are the contract provisions between a sponsor, investigator, and site for the conduct of a clinical trial.

Contract research organizations (CROs) refer to intermediary companies that provide sponsors with access to hospitals, physicians, and patients. These organizations largely contract directly with physicians outside of academic settings.

Clinical investigator refers to the physician responsible to the sponsor for the conduct of the clinical trial at the clinical trial site.

Subject means the patient involved in a clinical trial who will 'bear the risks of the research.'[113]

Academic Health Science Centre (AHSC) refers to a university, its medical school, and the teaching hospitals who agree to have collective action for a mission of excellence in education, research, and clinical care.

Table 6.1: Examples of the types of conflict of interest in industry-sponsored pre-approval clinical drug trials

	Main type of conflict	Examples
AHSC – Institution	Generating revenue for reinvestment into other hospital programs to sustain hospital mission	Hospital overhead charges for administering a trial
		Accepting donations, bonuses, etc. from the sponsor
	Attracting industry donors for clinical services and/or AHSC's research and educational programs	Obtaining reimbursement from the sponsor for usual (insured) care in a drug trial
		Altering usual approach to management of clinical trials to secure a donation from that sponsor
AHSC – Investigators	Generating revenue from clinical trial activity for the hospital, subspecialty group, or clinical service	Accepting bonuses or other financial rewards for patient recruitment in a clinical trial and/or for patient completion of the trial
	Generating personal income	Inflating the cost of services rendered in a clinical trial to generate a surplus for other academic purposes
	Conducting and publishing clinical trials that contribute to academic advancement	
		Allowing a sponsor to prepare a manuscript ('ghost-authorship')
		Altered management of clinical trials to increase sponsored research activity and/or publishing activity and/or secure donations
Non-AHSC investigators and their settings	Generating revenue from clinical trial activity for the hospital, subspecialty group, or clinical service	Accepting bonuses or other financial rewards for patient recruitment in a clinical trial and/or for patient completion of the trial
	Generating personal income	Inflating the cost of services rendered in a clinical trial
Journals	Generating advertising revenue	Publishing sponsored supplements or proceedings of industry-sponsored symposia without appropriate peer review
		Preferential publication of positive clinical trials to maintain advertising revenue
		Avoidance of commentaries and editorials critical of pharmaceutical products and companies to maintain relationships with potential advertisers

NOTES

1 'Sponsor' means an individual, corporate body, institution, or organization that conducts a clinical trial. *Food and Drug Regulations*, C.R.C., c. 870, Division 5 at C.05.001

2 See, e.g., Claire Turcotte Maatz, 'University Physician-Researcher Conflicts of Interest: The Inadequacy of Current Controls and Proposed Reform' (1992) 7 High Tech. L.J. 137; Erica Rose, 'Conflicts of Interest in Clinical Research: Legal and Ethical Issues: Financial Conflicts of Interest: How Are We Managing?' (2001) 8 Widener L. Symp. J. 1; Frances H. Miller, 'Symposium Trust Relationships Part 1 of 2: Trusting Doctors: Tricky Business When It Comes to Clinical Research' (2001) 81 B.U.L. Rev. 423; Michael J. Malinowski, 'Conflicts of Interest in Clinical Research: Legal and Ethical Issues: Institutional Conflicts and Responsibilities in an Age of Academic-Industry Alliances' (2001) 8 Widener L. Symp. J. 47; Annetine C. Gelijns and Samuel O. Thier, 'Medical Innovation and Institutional Interdependence: Rethinking University-Industry Connections' (2002) 287 J. Am. Med. Assoc. 72.

3 Thomas W. Merrill, 'Symposium: Beyond the Independent Counsel: Evaluating the Options' (1999) 43 Saint Louis U.L.J. 1047.

4 Dennis F. Thompson, 'Understanding Financial Conflicts of Interest' (1993) 329 New Eng. J. Med. 573.

5 See Patricia C. Kuszler, 'Curing Conflicts of Interest in Clinical Research: Impossible Dreams and Harsh Realities' (2001) 8 Widener L. Symp. J. 115, for a discussion of financial and non-financial conflicts of interest for individuals and institutions.

6 Jerome P. Kassirer and Marcia Angell, 'Financial Conflicts of Interest in Biomedical Research' (1993) 329 New Eng. J. Med. 570.

7 Marvin A. Konstam et al., 'A Device Is Not a Drug' (2003) 9 J. Cardiac Failure 155.

8 David Blumenthal, 'Biotech in Northeast Ohio Conference: Conflict of Interest in Biomedical Research' (2002) 12 Health Matrix 377.

9 See *Gelsinger v. Trustees of the Univ. of Pa.* (Phila. Cnty Ct. of C.P., 2000). The case was settled, so we do not know if the courts would have ruled that there was a failure to secure informed consent. 'Family Settles Suit over Teen's Death During Gene Therapy,' *Wall Street Journal*, 6 November 2000, B6.

10 See, e.g., Stephen E. Ronai, 'Growing Public Scrutiny of FDA Clinical Trials: Ethical and Regulatory Compliance to Avoid "Uninformed Consent" and Financial Conflicts of Interest' (2001) 65 Conn. Med. 661.

11 U.S., House Committee on Government Operations, *Are Scientific Misconduct and Conflicts of Interest Hazardous to Our Health?* (H.R. Doc. No. 688)

(Washington, DC: United States Government Printing Office, 1990) at 25 [*Scientific Misconduct*]. See Maatz, 'University Physician-Research Conflicts of Interest,' for a more in-depth discussion.

12 *Scientific Misconduct.*

13 Jeanne Lenzer, 'Alteplase for Stroke: Money and Optimistic Claims Buttress the "Brain Attack" Campaign' (2002) 324 Brit. Med. J. 723.

14 National Institute of Neurological Disorders and Stroke rt-PA Stroke Study Group, 'Tissue Plasminogen Activator for Acute Ischemic Stroke' (1995) 333 New Eng. J. Med. 1581.

15 Alvin Weinberg, 'Science and Its Limits: The Regulator's Dilemma,' in Chris Whipple, ed., *De Minimis Risk* (New York: Plenum Press, 1987), 27 at 37–8, who was referring to allowing unproveable associations or seriously flawed overestimations to emerge as serious social concerns, such as that of the connection between radiation and bodily harm. See Jeremy D. Frailberg and Michael J. Trebilcock, 'Risk Regulation: Technocratic and Democratic Tools for Regulatory Reform' (1998) 43 McGill L.J. 835, about the risks of over-regulation.

16 See Task Force on Academic Health Centres, *From Bench to Bedside: Preserving the Research Mission of Academic Health Centres: Findings and Recommendations of The Commonwealth Fund Task Force on Academic Health Centers* (New York: Commonwealth Fund, 1999).

17 See *University and Small Business Patent Procedure Act of 1980*, Pub. L. No. 96-517, § 6(a), 94 Stat. 3018 (35 U.S.C. 200 et seq.); *Stevenson-Wydler Technology Innovation Act of 1980*, Pub. L. No. 96–480, 94 Stat. 2311 (15 U.S.C. 3701 et seq.).

18 Lawrence O. Gostin and Michael O. Witt, 'Conflict of Interest Dilemmas in Biomedical Research' (1994) 271 J. Am. Med. Assoc. 547.

19 Industry Canada, *Canadian Industry Statistics: Data Tables, Pharmaceutical and Medicine Manufacturing* [North American Industry Classification System (NAICS) Code Number 32541], http://www.strategis.ic.gc.ca/canadian_industry_statistics/cis.ns f/IDE/cis32541defe.html.

20 The PMPRB, established in 1987 by amendments to the *Patent Act*, is an independent, federal, quasi-judicial board that regulates the prices of patented drugs.

21 Patented Medicine Prices Review Board, *Annual Report* (Ottawa: Patented Medicine Prices Review Board, 2002), http://www.pmprb.com/CMFiles/ar2002e21LEF-6252003–6142.pdf.

22 Ibid.

23 Industry Canada, *Canada's Biopharmaceutical Industry: Open for Global Business*, http://www/strategis.ic.gc.ca/SSG/ph01473e.html.

24 According to an Industry Canada report, the overall savings for conducting clinical trials in Canada can be as much as 45 per cent relative to the United States. The savings arise from our lower costs for labour, institutional overhead, diagnostic services, procedures, and therapeutic inventions. Moreover, Canada generally has lower payments to clinical investigators. Our CRO costs are also lower, with one case study showing that the Canadian per-diem monitoring fee was $US1,100, versus on average $US2,500 per day in the United States. See Government of Canada, *Clinical Trials in Canada: Quality with Cost Advantage. A Canada–United States Comparison* (Ottawa: Industry Canada, 2003).

25 As of 1 September 2001, all submissions received by TPD to investigate new drugs were reclassified by regulation as 'clinical trial applications.'

26 Health Canada, *Annual Drug Submission Performance 2002 Report*, Part 1, *Therapeutic Products Directorate (TPD)* (Ottawa: Health Canada, 2003).

27 Ibid.

28 *Food and Drugs Act*, R.S.C. 1985, c. F-27, s. 1.

29 In 1997, Health Canada began conducting a comprehensive review of its health protection legislation that would result in a proposal to replace the *Food and Drugs Act*, the *Hazardous Products Act*, the *Quarantine Act*, and the *Radiation Emitting Devices Act* with a *Canada Health Protection Act*. Two sets of consultations occurred, in the fall of 1998 and spring 2004. The proposed act is expected to be presented to Parliament in 2004. See http://www.hc-sc.gc.ca/hpfb-dgpsa/ocapi-bpcp/shared_responsibilities_tc_e.html.

 On 8 October 8th 2004, the Goverment of Canada introduced a new *Quarantine Act*: Bill C-12, *An act to prevent the introduction and spread of communicable diseases*, as they recognized the importance of moving forward on updating the Quarantine Act before 2005, 1st Sess. 38th Parl., 2004.

30 *Food and Drug Regulations*, see note 1 above.

31 Biological and radiopharmaceutical drugs are regulated by Health Canada's Biologics and Genetic Therapies Directorate and will not be discussed in this chapter. Medical devices are also not discussed.

32 Pursuant to the *Food and Drug Regulations*, C.05.005, C.05.006.

33 International Conference on Harmonisation (ICH) of Technical Requirements for Registration of Pharmaceuticals for Human Use, 'Good Clinical Practice: Consolidated Guideline,' http://www.ncehr-cnerh.org/english/gcp/; *Food and Drug Regulations*, C.05.010.

34 After a drug is given market authorization, it may still be the subject of a clinical trial. Phase IV clinical trials (post-marketing or surveillance studies) are conducted after a drug is approved. These studies obtain information about the long-term efficacy and toxicity of the marketed drugs.

35 'Extent to which a specific intervention, procedure, regimen or service provides a beneficial result under ideal conditions.' John M. Last, *A Dictionary of Epidemiology*, 3rd ed. (Oxford: Oxford University Press, 1995), *s.v.* 'efficacy.'

36 Food and Drug Regulations, c.05.001.

37 See, e.g., Lorraine E. Ferris, 'Industry-Sponsored Pharmaceutical Trials and Research Ethics Boards: Are They Cloaked in Too Much Secrecy?' (2002) 166 Can. Med. Assoc. J. 1279.

38 Michael McDonald, ed., *The Governance of Health Research Involving Human Subjects* (Ottawa: Law Commission of Canada, 2000). At this time, only Quebec has legislation regulating human subjects research (Art. 21 C.C.Q).

39 See Bernard M. Dickens, 'Governance Relations in Biomedical Research,' in McDonald, ed., *The Governance of Health Research Involving Human Subjects*, § C-1.

40 See, e.g., The Interagency Advisory Panel on Research Ethics (PRE), *Process and Principles for Developing a Canadian Governance System for the Ethical Conduct of Research Involving Humans* (April 2002), http://www.pre.ethics .gc.ca/english/policyinitiatives/governance01.cfm; National Council on Ethics in Human Research, *The Final Report of the Task Force on Accreditation* (March 2002), http://www.ncehr-cnerh.org/downloads/ FIN_TaskForceReport_EN.pdf; Social Sciences and Humanities Research Council, Standing Committee on Ethics and Integrity, *Public Assurance System for Research Involving Humans in Council-Funded Institutions* (August 2001), http://www.sshrc.ca/web/about/policies/PAS_e.pdf.

41 Science Advisory Board, Health Canada, 'A Canadian System of Oversight for the Governance of Research Involving Human Subjects' (February 2002), http://www.hc-sc.gc.ca/sab-ccs/feb2002_governance _subject_e.pdf. This document talks about accrediting REBs and establishing policies and structures for their regulation. It also acknowledges the 'common rule' which is recognized by approximately twenty U.S. federal departments and agencies. See Jennifer A. Henderson and John J. Smith, 'Financial Conflict of Interest in Medical Research: Overview and Analysis of Federal and State Controls' (2002) 57 Food & Drug L.J. 445, for a description of the American 'common rule.'

42 See, e.g., 21 C.F.R. § 54. See also Guidance for Industry on Financial Disclosure by Clinical Investigators, http://222.fda.gov/oc/guidance/ financialdis.html.

43 In December 2002, the authors wrote to the Health Products and Food Branch Inspectorate (Registered as 02–121179-994) regarding their inspection strategy for clinical trials in human subjects. The letter is available at

www.library.utoronto.ca/medicine/medUT/hcletter.pdf. Health Canada's response to this letter is also available: www.library.utoronto.ca/medicine/medUT/lettresp.pdf. In our letter, we indicated that they could play a role in monitoring clinical trials for COI through their current regulatory framework. Our letter identified four main areas for improvement: (1) no physician financial incentive to recruit patients or for the successful completion of the trial; (2) no inappropriate inducements to investigators or to sites for their participation in a trial; (3) freedom of investigators to communicate directly and without delay or censorship to our regulatory system if there is a discontinuance of a clinical trial and their site or if there are serious unexpected study-related adverse events; and (4) freedom of investigators to communicate directly and without delay or censorship to the scientific community. This would require the review, during site visits, of clinical trial agreements, the investigators' brochure for the drug, and any related financial agreements. Health Canada said that these suggestions fell outside the scope of Division 5 of the inspection program. With respect to point (3), Health Canada said that qualified investigators may report on the discontinuation of a clinical trial (C.05.015) and serious unexpected adverse drug reactions (C.05.014) under the Regulations, although sponsors have the legislative responsibility to do so.

44 See the TPD, Policy Division, Bureau of Policy and Coordination concerning the Regulations Amending the Food and Drug Regulations, *Regulatory Impact Analysis Statement, (1024 Clinical Trials)* at 22, http://www.hc-sc.gc.ca/hpfb-dgpsa/inspectorate/food_drug_reg_amend_1024_gcp_e.pdf.

45 Division 5 in the *Food and Drug Regulations* concerns 'Drugs for Clinical Trials Involving Human Subjects.'

46 Health Products and Food Branch Inspectorate, *Summary Report of the Inspections of Clinical Trials Conducted under Voluntary Phase* (July 2003), http://www.hc-sc.gc.ca/hpfb-dgpsa/inspectorate/gcp_inspection_sum_rep_entire_e.html.

47 Ibid.

48 Jeffrey C. Lozon and Robert M. Fox, 'Academic Health Sciences Centres Laid Bare' (2002) 2:3 Healthcare Papers 10.

49 There is a tension between universities/medical schools and the teaching hospitals about education and patient care. The university/medical school may decide to increase or decrease medical student or post-graduate enrolment (and how and where these trainees will be assigned for their clinical experience), affecting the teaching hospitals' patient care program. Similarly, hospitals may decrease or eliminate a program, add a new program,

or move to a different patient care model, affecting the university/medical schools' education program.

50 See, e.g., Richard Culbertson, 'A U.S. Perspective: A Future of Increased Diversification' (2002) 2:3 Healthcare Papers 66.

51 Lozon and Fox, 'Academic Health Sciences Centres Laid Bare.'

52 See, e.g., Michael A. Weber, 'Impact on the Pharmaceutical Industry of Changes in the American Health Care System: A Physician's Perspective' (1994) 24 Seton Hall L. Rev. 1290.

53 See, e.g., Patricia C. Kuszler, 'Financial Clinical Research and Experimental Therapies: Payment Due, But From Whom?' (2000) 3 DePaul J. Health Care L. 441, for a discussion of this issue. Henry J. Aaron and Hellen Gelband, eds., *Extending Medicare Reimbursement in Clinical Trials* (Washington, DC: National Academy Press, 2000), says the revenue may in part come from being reimbursed in a clinical trial for usual care where there are already provisions for reimbursement of it.

54 See, e.g., Bryan J. Weiner et al., 'Organizational Models for Medical School-Clinical Enterprise Relationships' (2001) 76 Acad. Med. 113; Jay K. Levine, 'Considering Alternative Organizational Structures for Academic Medical Centers' (2002) 14:2 Acad. Clinical Practice 2.

55 The American Association of University Professors has published the original statements about academic freedom with their 1970 interpretive comments and policies concerning academic freedom in one report, referred to as the 'Redbook.' *1940 Statement of Principles on Academic Freedom and Tenure with 1970 Interpretive Comments*, http://www.aaup.org/statements/Redbook/1940stat.htm.

56 C. David Naylor, 'The CMA's First Code of Ethics: Medical Morality or Borrowed Ideology?' (1983) 17:4 J. Can. Stud. 20.

57 *Dickason v. University of Alberta*, [1992], 2 S.C.R. 1103. See also *Students for Life v. Alma Mater Society of the University of British Columbia* (2003), 15 B.C.L.R. (4th) 358 (S.C.).

58 *McKinney v. University of Guelph*, [1990] 3 S.C.R. 229 at 286–7, 376.

59 See Canadian Association of University Teachers, *Policy Statement on Academic Freedom* (May 2003), http://www.caut.ca/English/about/policy/academic freedom.asp.

60 Rebecca S. Eisenberg, 'Symposium on Academic Freedom: Academic Freedom and Academic Values in Sponsored Research' (1988) 66 Tex. L. Rev. 1363.

61 See, e.g., David G. Nathan and David J. Weatherall, 'Academic Freedom in Clinical Research' (2002) 347 New Eng. J. Med. 1368; Jeffrey M. Drazen, 'Institutions, Contracts, and Academic Freedom' (2002) 347 New Eng. J.

Med. 1362. For a discussion about systemic reforms addressing issues in contract research conducted at academic health sciences centres, see Lorraine E. Ferris, Peter A. Singer, and C. David Naylor, 'Better Governance in Academic Health Sciences Centres: Moving Beyond the Olivieri/Apotex Affair in Toronto' (2004) 30 J. Med. Ethics 25.

62 See Richard A. Deyo et al., 'The Messenger under Attack: Intimidation of Researchers by Special-Interest Groups' (1997) 336 New Eng. J. Med. 1176.

63 See Association of American Universities, Task Force on Research Accountability, *Report on Individual and Institutional Financial Conflict of Interest* (October 2001), http://www.aau.edu/research/COI.01.pdf.

64 Brenda L. Beagan, 'Ethics Review for Human Subjects Research: Interviews with Members of Research Ethics Boards and National Organizations,' in McDonald, ed., *The Governance of Health Research Involving Human Subjects*, § E-1.

65 Government of Canada, *Clinical Trials in Canada*.

66 Frank Davidoff et al., 'Sponsorship, Authorship and Accountability' (2001) 135 Annals Internal Med. 463.

67 Thomas Bodenheimer, 'Uneasy Alliance: Clinical Investigators and the Pharmaceutical Industry' (2000) 342 New Eng. J. Med. 1539. See also Gelijns and Thier, 'Medical Innovation and Institutional Interdependence.'

68 See Kenneth A. Getz, *AMCs Rekindling Clinical Research Partnerships with Industry* (Boston: Centerwatch, 1999); Task Force on Academic Health Centres, *From Bench to Bedside*.

69 See Stephen Zisson, 'Losing Ground in the Battle against Development Delays' (1998) 5:12 CenterWatch 1 at 1, 3.

70 CenterWatch, 'Pace of CRO Acquisitions Accelerates' (2002) 9:7 CenterWatch 1.

71 Covance Inc. et al., Letter to the Editor, 'Sponsorship, Authorship, and Accountability' (2000) 136 Annals Internal Med. 251.

72 See Karine Morin et al., 'Managing Conflicts of Interest in the Conduct of Clinical Trials' (2002) 287 J. Am. Med. Assoc. 78.

73 Ibid.

74 See Trudo Lemmens and Benjamin Freedman, 'Ethics Review for Sale?' (2000) 78 Milbank Q. 547.

75 See Jonathan Quick, 'Maintaining the Integrity of the Clinical Evidence Base' (2001) 79 Bulletin of the World Health Organization 1093, who argues that for such progress to continue there needs to be a declaration on the 'rights and obligations of clinical investigators and on how to manage the entire clinical trials evidence base' in a similar initiative as the *Helsinki Dec-*

laration that addressed the unacceptable risk to research subjects in research studies.

76 Several editorials in medical journals have addressed this issue. See, e.g., Marcia Angell, 'Is Academic Medicine for Sale?' (2000) 342 New Eng. J. Med. 1516; Martin B. Van Der Weyden, 'Confronting Conflict of Interest in Research Organisations: Time for National Action' (2001) 175 Med. J. Aus. 396; Catherine D. DeAngelis, 'Conflict of Interest and the Public Trust' (2001) 284 J. Am. Med. Assoc. 2237; John F. Staropoli, 'Funding and Practice of Biomedical Research' (2003) 290 J. Am. Med. Assoc. 112; and 'The Controlling Interests of Research' Editorial (2002) 167 Can. Med. Assoc. J. 1221.

77 See, e.g., David Korn, 'Conflicts of Interest in Biomedical Research' (2000) 284 J. Am. Med. Assoc. 2234; Niteesh K. Choudhry, Henry Thomas Stelfox, and Allan S. Detsky, 'Relationships between Authors of Clinical Practice Guidelines and the Pharmaceutical Industry' (2002) 287 J. Am. Med. Assoc. 612; Charles Warlow, 'Who Pays the Guideline Writers?' (2002) 324 Brit. Med. J. 726; and Lisa A. Bero and Drummond Rennie, 'Influences on the Quality of Published Drug Studies' (1996) 12 Int'l J. Tech. Assessment Health Care 209.

78 See, e.g., Patricia Baird, 'Getting It Right: Industry Sponsorship and Medical Research' (2003) 168 Can. Med. Assoc. J. 1267; Gelijns and Thier, 'Medical Innovation and Institutional Interdependence'; Paul S. Thomas, Ken-Soon Tan, and Deborah H. Yates, 'Sponsorship, Authorship, and Accountability' Letter (2002) 359 Lancet 351; Henry Thomas Stelfox et al., 'Conflict of Interest in the Debate over Calcium-Channel Antagonists' (1998) 338 New Eng. J. Med. 101; and Mark Friedberg et al., 'Evaluation of Conflict of Interest in Economic Analyses of New Drugs Used in Oncology' (1999) 282 J. Am. Med. Assoc. 1453.

79 Some view the premature termination of clinical trials for economic reasons rather than for ethical or scientific reasons as a violation of the *Declaration of Helsinki* because it may not be in the best interests of research subjects. See, e.g., Bruce M. Psaty and Drummond Rennie, 'Stopping Medical Research to Save Money: A Broken Pact with Researchers and Patients' (2003) 289 J. Am. Med. Assoc. 2128; Kenneth Boyd, 'Early Discontinuation Violates Helsinki Principles' (2001) 322 Brit. Med. J. 605. See also Michel Lièvre et al., 'Premature Discontinuation of Clinical Trial for Reasons Not Related to Efficacy, Safety, or Feasibility' (2001) 322 Brit. Med. J. 603. However, as Eric P. Brass has pointed out in 'Premature Termination of Clinical Trials' (2003) 290 J. Am. Med. Assoc. 595, this is a problem for investigator-initiated studies as well.

80 See, e.g., David Blumenthal et al., 'Withholding Research Results in Aca-

demic Life Science: Evidence from a National Survey of Faculty' (1997) 277 J. Am. Med. Assoc. 1224; Iain Chalmers, 'Underreporting Research Is Scientific Misconduct' (1990) 263 J. Am. Med. Assoc. 1405; Drummond Rennie, 'Thyroid Storm' (1997) 277 J. Am. Med. Assoc. 1238; Bodenheimer, 'Uneasy Alliance'; Robert A. Phillips and John Hoey, 'Constraints of Interest: Lessons at the Hospital for Sick Children' (1998) 159 Can. Med. Assoc. J. 955; and Jerome M. Stern and R. John Simes, 'Publication Bias: Evidence of Delayed Publication in a Cohort Study of Clinical Research Projects' (1997) 315 Brit. Med. J. 640.

81 See, e.g., Bero and Rennie, 'Influences on the Quality of Published Drug Studies'; Joel Lexchin et al., 'Pharmaceutical Industry Sponsorship and Research Outcome and Quality: Systematic Review' (2003) 326 Brit. Med. J. 326; Paula A. Rochon et al., 'A Study of Manufacturer-Supported Trials of Nonsteroidal Anti-Inflammatory Drugs in the Treatment of Arthritis' (1994) 154 Arch. Internal Med. 157; Justin E. Bekelman, Yan Li, and Cary P. Gross, 'Scope and Impact of Financial Conflicts of Interest in Biomedical Research: A Systematic Review' (2003) 289 J. Am. Med. Assoc. 454; Philippa J. Easterbrook et al., 'Publication Bias in Clinical Research' (1991) 337 Lancet 867; Kay Dickersin, Simon Chan, and Thomas C. Chalmers, 'Publication Bias and Clinical Trials' (1987) 8 Controlled Clinical Trials 343; Richard A. Davidson, 'Source of Funding and Outcome of Clinical Trials' (1986) 1 J. Gen. Internal Med. 155; and Mildred K. Cho and Lisa A. Bero, 'The Quality of Drug Studies Published in Symposium Proceedings' (1996) 124 Annals Internal Med. 485. In a revealing *British Medical Journal* editorial, Richard Smith has addressed the issue of journal supplements and the poorer scientific quality of these clinical trials. He says these are a major profit-making initiative for the journal. See Richard Smith, 'Medical Journals and Pharmaceutical Companies: Uneasy Bedfellows' (2003) 326 Brit. Med. J. 1202. See also Drummond Rennie, 'Fair Conduct and Fair Reporting of Clinical Trials' (1999) 282 J. Am. Med. Assoc. 1766, who discusses, among other things, the problem of redundant publication in reporting clinical trial results, and the belief that these duplicate trial publications had results in favour of the sponsor. See Hans Melander et al., 'Evidence B(i)ased Medicine: Selective Reporting From Studies Sponsored by Pharmaceutical Industry: Review of Studies in New Drug Applications' (2003) 326 Brit. Med. J. 1171, where the authors documented multiple publication, selective publication, and selective reporting of placebo controlled studies involving serotonin reuptake inhibitors. Iain Chalmers, 'Underreporting Research is Scientific Misconduct,' says that many of those involved in clinical trials (i.e., investigators, research ethics boards, funding bodies, and scientific editors) have a

responsibility to reduce underreporting of clinical trials since the failure to publish is a form of scientific misconduct.

82 See, e.g., Arnold S. Relman, 'Dealing with Conflicts of Interest' (1984) 310 New Eng. J. Med. 1182; Marcia Angell, Robert D. Utiger, and Alastair J.J. Wood, 'Disclosure of Authors' Conflicts of Interest: A Follow-Up' (2002) 342 New Eng. J. Med. 586; Drummond Rennie, Annette Flanagin, and Richard M. Glass, 'Conflicts of Interest in the Publication of Science' (1991) 266 J. Am. Med. Assoc. 266; and Richard Smith, 'Conflict of Interest and the BMJ' (1994) 308 Brit. Med. J. 4.

83 S. Van McCrary et al., 'A National Survey of Policies on Disclosure of Conflicts of Interest in Biomedical Research' (2000) 343 New Eng. J. Med. 1621.

84 Sheldon Krimsky and Leslie S. Rothenberg, 'Conflict of Interest Policies and Science and Medical Journals: Editorial Practices and Author Disclosures' (2001) 7 Sci. Engineering Ethics 205.

85 For a brief overview see Fran Van Kolfschooten, 'Conflicts of Interest: Can You Believe What You Read?' (2002) 416 Nature 360.

86 'Ghost writing' is a concern, since it may conceal financial COI. It allows other authors to take credit for the work, and fails to recognize those meeting the criteria for eligible authors. See, e.g., Marilynn Larkin, 'Whose Article Is it Anyway?' (1999) 354 Lancet 136; Drummond Rennie and Annette Flanagin, 'Authorship! Authorship! Guests, Ghosts, Grafters, and the Two-sided Coin' (1994) 271 J. Am. Med. Assoc. 469.

87 Davidoff et al., 'Sponsorship, Authorship and Accountability.' This same statement was published by other medical journals of which the editor participated in its writing.

88 Ibid. at 826.

89 Ibid. at 827.

90 International Committee of Medical Journal Editors, *Uniform Requirements for Manuscripts Submitted to Biomedical Journals: Writing and Editing for Biomedical Publication* (November 2003), http://www.icmje.org.

91 See Elizabeth Wager, 'How to Dance with Porcupines: Rules and Guidelines on Doctors' Relations with Drug Companies' (2003) 326 Brit. Med. J. 1196; Stanley G. Korenman, 'The Role of Journal Editors in the Responsible Conduct of Industry-Sponsored Biomedical Research and Publication: A View from the Other Side of the Editor's Desk' (2003) 26 Science Editor 42.

92 See, e.g., Hiram C. Polk, Jr et al., 'Consensus Statement on Scientific Data from Clinical Trials and Investigators' Responsibilities and Rights' (2002) 183 Am. J. Surgery 605.

93 See Richard Smith, 'Maintaining the Integrity of the Scientific Record' (2001) 323 Brit. Med. J. 588.

94 See Lawrence J. Hirsch, 'Conflicts of Interest in Drug Development: The Practices of Merck & Co., Inc.' (2002) 8 Sci. Engineering Ethics 429; Pharmaceutical Research and Manufacturers of America, *Principles on Conduct of Clinical Trials and Communication of Clinical Trial Results* (July 2002), http://www.phrma.org/publications/policy/2002-07-18.490.pdf. See also Elizabeth Wager, Elizabeth A. Field, and Leni Grossman, 'Good Publication Practice for Pharmaceutical Companies' (2003) 19 Curr. Med. Research Opinion 149, which provides guidelines from industry concerning good publication practices of clinical trials. Although these are progressive, they do endorse the use of medical writers and only six of seventy-five pharmaceutical companies endorsed them (see Debashis Singh, 'Drug Companies Advised to Publish Unfavourable Trial Results' (2003) 326 Brit. Med. J. 1163).

95 There have been several initiatives in this area. As early as 1995, the American Bar Association (ABA) and the American Law Institute (ALI) held a continuing legal education course on biotechnology (business, law, and regulation) that included a subsection on clinical trials and clinical trial agreements (co-sponsored by California Continuing Education of the Bar). See Charlotte H. Harrison, 'Clinical Trials: Contracting with Institutions and Investigators – Practical and Policy Issues from an Institution's Perspective' (1995) 3 ALI-ABA 9. This paper also presented a draft clinical trial agreement. In 2002 the Association of American Medical Colleges (AAMC) established a PhRMA/AAMC Forum which discusses issues concerning industry-sponsored trials, enhances communication and collaboration between academic institutions and sponsors, and tries to improve the quality of industry-sponsored trials in academic settings. The pharmaceutical companies that participate include Aventis, Lilly, Merck, Pfizer, P&G, and PhRMA; the academic sites include the AAMC, Columbia University, Johns Hopkins University, Northwestern University, UCLA, and Washington University. Since the beginning of the forum, issues such as contract approval process, publication of data, and use of central IRBs by academia have been discussed. In July 2003 the forum discussed, among other things, the language of contracts. See 'Addressing the Issues: Academic and Industry Perspectives on Clinical Trials' (A Conference Sponsored by AAMC and PhRMA and the PhRMA/AAMC Forum, 10 July 2003).

96 Kevin A. Schulman et al., 'A National Survey of Provisions in Clinical-Trial Agreements between Medical Schools and Industry Sponsors' (2002) 347 New Eng. J. Med. 1335.

97 In November 2002, a *Canadian Medical Association Journal* editorial suggested that the study by Kevin A. Schulman et al. be replicated in Canada.

See 'The Controlling Interests of Research' Editorial (2002) 167 Can. Med. Assoc. J. 1221. The Canadian Institutes of Health Research recently announced a call for proposals in this area.

98 C. David Naylor, 'Early Toronto Experience with New Standards for Industry-Sponsored Clinical Research: A Progress Report' (2002) 166 Can. Med. Assoc. J. 453.

99 In late 2002, the Toronto Academic Health Sciences Centre expanded these three principles to include, among other things: the right of investigators to retain a copy of data gathered at their site; the right to publish or present on single-site results if a publication is not prepared for the multi-site trial; disclosure to study subjects, sponsor, study steering committee, research ethics boards at the site, and other participating sites and regulators, if and when the investigation (institution and/or REB) deem that disclosure is necessary to protect the health of student participants; and no binding arbitration of disagreements between the sponsor and the investigator on matters related to patient safety. These principles were embedded in the affiliation agreement between the university and its fully affiliated teaching hospitals.

100 See Association of American Medical Colleges, Task Force on Financial Conflicts of Interest in Clinical Research, *Protecting Subjects, Preserving Trust, Promoting Progress II: Principles and Recommendations for Oversight of an Institution's Financial Interests in Human Subjects Research* (October 2002), http://www.aamc.org/members/coitf/2002coireport.pdf; Association of American Medical Colleges, Task Force on Financial Conflicts of Interest in Clinical Research, *Protecting Subjects, Preserving Trust, Promoting Progress – Policy and Guidelines for the Oversight of Individual Financial Interest in Human Subjects Research* (December 2001), www.aamc.org/members/coitf/firstreport.pdf.

101 Association of American Universities, Task Force on Research Accountability, *Report on Individual and Institutional Financial Conflict of Interest.*

102 See, e.g., American Association of University Professors, Committee on Academic Freedom and Tenure, *Statement on Corporate Funding of Academic Research* (May 2001), http://www.aaup.org/statements/Redbook/repcorf.htm.

103 See, e.g., Bernardine Healy et al., 'Conflict of Interest Guidelines for a Multicenter Clinical Trial of Treatment after Coronary-Artery Bypass-Graft Surgery' (1989) 320 New Eng. J. Med. 949; Eric J. Topol et al., 'Confronting the Issues of Patient Safety and Investigator Conflict of Interest in an International Clinical Trial of Myocardial Reperfusion' (1992) 19 J. Am. College Cardiology 1123.

104 Academic freedom has collective as well as individual aspects. See *Re University of Calgary and University of Calgary Faculty Association*, [1999] C.L.A.S.J. LEXIS 4051.

105 Peter J. Harrington, 'Faculty Conflicts of Interest in an Age of Academic Entrepreneurialism: An Analysis of the Problem, the Law and Selected University Policies' (2001) 27 J.C. & U.L. 774.

106 Ibid.

107 See Bernard Lo, Leslie E. Wolf, and Abiona Berkeley, 'Conflict of Interest Policies for Investigators in Clinical Trials' (2000) 343 New Eng. J. Med. 1616; Van McCrary et al., 'National Survey of Policies on Disclosure of Conflicts of Interest'; Mildred K. Cho et al., 'Policies on Faculty Conflicts of Interest at U.S. Universities' (2000) 284 J. Am. Med. Assoc. 2203. In this study, only 19 per cent of policies had clear limits on the financial interests of faculty in corporate sponsors.

108 See, e.g., Cho et al., 'Policies on Faculty Conflicts of Interest.'

109 See, e.g., Debra Blum, 'Universities, Researchers Struggle to Develop Policies Aimed at Avoiding Potential Conflicts of Interest' (1990) 36:33 Chronicle Higher Ed. 33.

110 The chapter authors have since written about the need for standardized clinical trial budgets. See Lorraine E. Ferris and C. David Naylor, 'Physician Remuneration in Industry-sponsored Clinical Trials: The Case for Standardized Clinical Trial Budgets' (2004) 171 Can. Med. Assoc. J. 883; and Lorraine E. Ferris and C. David Naylor, 'Rebuttal' (2004) 171 Can. Med. Assoc. J. 892.

111 Dennis F. Thompson, 'Understanding Financial Conflicts of Interest' (1993) 329 New England J. Med. 573.

112 *Food and Drug Regulations*, C.05.001.

113 See Medical Research Council of Canada, Natural Sciences and Engineering Research Council of Canada, and the Social Sciences and Humanities Research Council of Canada, *Tri-Council Policy Statement: Ethical Conduct for Research Involving Humans* (Ottawa: Public Works and Government Services Canada, 1998), http://www.pre.ethics.gc.ca/english/policystatement/policystateme nt.cfm.

7 The Human Subjects Trade: Ethical, Legal, and Regulatory Remedies to Deal with Recruitment Incentives and to Protect Scientific Integrity

TRUDO LEMMENS AND PAUL B. MILLER

Over the past five years, a series of articles in leading American newspapers has revealed the extent to which the conduct of clinical trials may be affected by inducements offered by corporate research sponsors and accepted by some unscrupulous physicians.[1] The cases described were disturbing. They involved physicians engaged in excessive 'enrolment activities' in exchange for money. Some of these physicians perpetrated fraud, falsifying their recruitment records in order to increase their profits. Others ignored exclusion criteria designed to ensure the safety of subjects and the validity of research results, referring their patients to research investigating treatments for conditions from which they did not suffer.[2] One of the articles reports that physicians focusing exclusively on commercial research regularly divulge annual incomes upwards of $1 million with profits in excess of $300,000. Two physicians accumulated well over $10 million through clinical trials activities in less than a decade.[3] Another article reported the role of finder's fees and payments to parents in increasing the enrolment of children in medical research in the United States from 16,000 in 1997 to 45,000 in 2001.[4] It also highlighted the fact that subjects may be exposed to serious harm through referrals by zealous and inexperienced physicians, drawn to recruitment activity by offers of up to $5,000 per patient referred. Finally, several other 'disturbing recruitment practices' were reported by the U.S. Department of Health and Human Services' Office of Inspector General in its report on subject recruitment practices. These include many cases of patients being harassed for participation; a nursing home resident being told to participate in research or leave the home; and a subject who died and was later found not to have met the inclusion criteria for the study.[5]

Because of their arguably extreme nature, and the fact that regulatory agencies did eventually intervene, these cases could all too easily be brushed aside as the exceptional dirty laundry in an otherwise clean research environment. The rather limited analysis and discussion of finder's fees in the literature[6] may both reflect and reinforce the unwarranted belief that they are rare and adequately dealt with under existing professional and research ethics codes and policies. Offers of finder's fees ranging between two and five thousand dollars per subject are now regarded as 'common' in the United States.[7] The lack of similar reports in other countries could give the impression that finder's fees raise troubling issues only in the United States. This is not the case. We have heard personal testimony from various sources in Canada indicating that many Canadian physicians and other health care workers receive up to several thousands of dollars for enrolling patients in, or referring them to, clinical trials. Direct evidence of this practice, is unfortunately, hard to obtain. Those involved have no interest in drawing attention to their activities, and their colleagues are understandably reluctant to speak out.

We believe that the issues surrounding finder's fees and other recruitment incentives merit more careful scrutiny. The payment of finder's fees for subject recruitment can be seen as a paradigmatic example of other problematic phenomena in an increasingly commercial research environment. When situated within this context, it becomes clear that the actual and potential impact of finder's fees is more significant than has been presumed. The problems resulting from finder's fees are part of the wider encroachment of commercial interests on research, the provision of health care services, and the priorities of researchers and health care professionals. These issues ought to receive more attention from regulatory and funding agencies, professional organizations, academic institutions, Institutional Review Boards (IRBs) – known in Canada as Research Ethics Boards (REBs) – and researchers. Representatives of each of these interests have an important role to play in addressing the tensions generated by financial interests in research.

There are significant problems with the mechanisms by which conflicts of interest are currently managed and governed. In our view, finder's fees and other controversial issues in research have often been dealt with in isolation, and in a way sheltered from analyses that would open up the possibility of 'legal interference.' Discussions about finder's fees and other recruitment incentives are often oriented solely by reference to institutional, national, and international ethics guidelines. They remain curiously silent on the parties' legal obligations and potential legal sanctions. This reflects and encourages inordinate reliance on the overly general conflicts of interest rules in ethics guidelines, and on the inadequately regulated American (or largely unregulated Canadian) system of IRB/REB review. Some legislated standards of professional conduct and court rulings provide much more stringent benchmarks for the behaviour of physicians in research, but these have been largely ignored and inadequately enforced. This paper aims to create awareness of the seriousness of the issues surrounding finder's fees, and to detail relevant ethical, legal, and policy standards. We argue that stricter oversight of conflicts of interest by institutional and regulatory authorities, and better enforcement of existing regulatory and legal remedies are needed to safeguard the rights and well-being of research subjects and to preserve the integrity of the medical profession and the research process. In addition, we point out that instances of concealed profiteering from research recruitment activities could attract criminal sanctions. This alone highlights the importance of professional organizations and funding and regulatory agencies turning their full attention to the development of adequate controls for recruitment activities.

Finder's Fees in Context

Finder's fees are offers of money to physicians, nurses, or other health professionals in reward for their referral of patients eligible for research participation (i.e., they represent payment for referrals, over and above reasonable remuneration for services rendered). The general view on finder's fees as reflected in various ethics guidelines is straightforward: they are deemed unacceptable. That said, finder's fees are in reality rarely clearly indicated as such. They are instead most often integrated into the budgets of clinical trials, usually described only as payment of 'administrative costs.' Since existing guidelines generally allow researchers and research personnel to be compensated for extra time spent on research, finder's fees can easily be hidden among bona fide expenses. Moreover, significant incentives can be independent of what is provided through the budget of a trial, and thereby doubly hard to directly associate with the recruitment of subjects. Researchers who have been successful in recruiting patients may, for example, be rewarded not with fees, but with equally valuable invitations to make well-paid presentations of research findings, or to participate in prestigious seminars at interesting locations.[8] Financial interests and concomitant feelings of obligation to sponsors can also be generated through the appointment of researchers to lucrative positions on sponsors' scientific advisory boards and specialized committees, or through paid consulting relationships.[9] Strong sponsorship ties between researchers, research institutions, and industry may also come with the pressure of sponsors' expectations of better access to the patient populations of the institution.

Whether or not express, finder's fees are now commonplace, and are but one indication of the increasingly competitive environment in which contract research organizations (CROs), academic research institutes, and pharmaceutical companies compete for access to research subjects.[10] The increased demand and competition for subjects is a reflection of the spectacular increase in research activity over the last two decades, an increase in large part driven by growing commercial interest in research. The forces generated by increasing commercial investment in research are particularly apparent in the context of clinical trials focusing on drug development.

Recent publications have detailed elements of the overall context within which finder's fees ought to be understood.[11] We can touch only briefly upon these elements presently. A PriceWaterhouseCoopers report has suggested that in order to maintain levels of profitability, pharmaceuticals companies will have to launch, on average, between twenty-four and thirty-four new drugs per year.[12] This in part explains why, as of 1999, more than 450 medicines were under development for heart disease, cancer, and stroke, and why a further 191 were being developed for Alzheimer's, arthritis, and depression.[13] This also explains in part the surge in numbers of physicians involved in clinical trials: 30,000 more physicians were involved in clinical trials in the United States in 1998 than a decade earlier, an increase of 600 per cent.[14] Over the same period, there has been 60 per cent increase in numbers of community-based clinical trials conducted.[15] As the latter data indicate, community-based physicians, most often remunerated through monetary incentives, are increasingly competing with researchers in academic institutions for access to research subjects.[16] The conduct of clinical trials is shifting from the teaching hospitals of academic institutions to the offices of private physicians and CROs.[17]

How the above-noted trends translate in terms of numbers of subjects enrolled per annum in research can unfortunately only be guessed at. No official numbers are available in the United States or Canada. This in itself is an indication of the troubling lacunae in the oversight of research. In order to understand the importance of regulation and oversight, as well as the human significance of existing pressures on the system, it is surely essential that we know how many people participate in research. Adil E. Shamoo has estimated – based on U.S. National Institutes of Health (NIH) data on expenditures per subject and available statistics on gross private investment in research – that approximately 18 million people participate in research each year in the United States, which amounts to approximately 6 per cent of the total population.[18]

No estimate has been made in Canada, and no official agency has figures upon which to base a reliable calculation. If Shamoo's estimate is reliable, and if a similar percentage of the Canadian population would participate in research, roughly 1,865,000 Canadians would participate as subjects in research each year.[19] This may seem an extremely high number, but there are sufficient indicators that it is closer to the truth than one would think, and that at least several hundred thousand of Canadians participate in research each year. Considering its limited population, Canada has a significant clinical trials industry and a vibrant research sector. Canada is situated third in numbers of clinical trials undertaken annually, after the United States and Europe. The Therapeutic Products Directorate of Health Canada has reported that there were eight hundred clinical trial submissions in Canada in 1998, and that it has witnessed an average 20 per cent annual increase in applications.[20] If this rate of increase has held steady, the Therapeutic Products Directorate would have received approximately 1,658 applications to conduct clinical trials in 2002. These clinical trials alone would require the enrolment of hundred thousands of people. A recent article indicates that Can$900 million is spent annually by pharmaceutical companies and CROs on inhouse research and development in Canada.[21] Industry further invests Can$161 million in Canadian universities and teaching hospitals.[22] Funding agencies, both federal and provincial, contributed close to Can$300 million.[23] The overall amount of approximately Can$1.36 billion compares with combined industry and government expenditures estimated at US$42 billion in the United States.[24]

These actual and estimated demographic trends are indicative of the advent of a highly competitive research environment. In this environment, research subjects have become a scarce and valuable commodity.[25] Pressure to recruit subjects exists not only because of the sheer number of trials being undertaken: the speed with which trials are conducted has significant financial implications as well. Where an experimental drug or device is expected to have considerable medical and market potential, corporate sponsors of research and researchers alike are under enormous pressure to ensure that the research is undertaken as efficiently as possible. Development costs of new medications have been estimated to range between $300 and $600 million in the United States.[26] Industry has argued that a one-day delay in getting a drug on the market comes with a price tag of $1.3 million.[27] Although some industry claims about costs of drug development are questionable and seem to function more as a tool to influence drug policies,[28] it is clear that delays in approval have financial repercussions.

Developments in pharmacogenomics may increase the demand for research subjects. Pharmacogenomics research investigates the role of genetics in drug response. Some predict that pharmacogenomic research will result in the fragmentation of conventional disease categories, in accordance with newly discovered patterns of genetic variation affecting drug response. If this prediction proves true, researchers may be required to conduct more focused trials on smaller targeted subpopulations to fulfil regulatory requirements.

For a trial to be efficient it must, among other things, produce valid results (further trials mean further costs). For a trial to produce valid results, sufficient numbers of subjects must be recruited, enrolled, and retained. Corporate sponsors work to ensure that sufficient numbers of subjects are enrolled through offering remuneration both to researchers and research subjects.[29] One executive of a U.S.-based CRO recently admitted that the pressure to recruit subjects has led corporate sponsors to enlist in recruitment activity 'anybody who has a population ... they are taking care of.'[30] Interviewed for the *Boston Globe*, Newell Unfried, vice-president of a group of leading for-profit research centres, stated that pharmaceuticals companies draw up performance reviews on patient recruitment of every physician involved in clinical research.[31] The Office of Inspector General has confirmed this and further reports that 'sponsors and their agents constantly remind sites of the need to expedite recruitment. Sites report numerous phone calls from sponsors, informing them of how their enrolment statistics compare with those of other sites in the trial.'[32]

According to one commentator, the shift to community-based research can be explained at least in part by the fact that community-based physicians 'have become a reliable source of patients.'[33] Realizing that there is money to be had for the referral of their patients to research, some community-based researchers have gone as far as to advertise the size of their patient base. The Office of Inspector General reports that one community-based practice placed an internet ad, reading in part as follows:

Looking for Trials!
We are a large family practice office ... We have two full time coordinators and a computerized patient data base of 40,000 patients ... We are looking for Phase 2–Phase 4 trials as well as postmarketing studies. We can actively recruit patients for any study that can be conducted in the Family Practice setting.[34]

The movement towards community-based research, often involving less qualified researchers, has the effect of further concentrating sponsors' power over trial design, subject selection, data collection, and interpretation of results.[35] Dr Sidney Wolfe, director of the Public Citizens' Health Research Group, has commented on the relationship between the increasing commercialization of research, offers of finder's fees, and the shift to community-based research as follows:

The number of private practice-based investigators has grown from 3153 in 1990 to 11588 in 1995, an increase of almost four-fold ... concomitant with the increasing domination of human experimentation corporations in experimentation. The vulnerability of a doctor's own patients to become an experimental research subject because of their trust in their doctor, combined with the signing bonuses, which the doctor pockets for the referral, sets up a toxic situation where some doctors are literally selling their own patients into human experiments.[36]

Unfortunately, cut-throat competition for research subjects has become widespread. We received various personal accounts of troubling recruitment practices in university-affiliated hospitals. One person, for example, told of a research coordinator trying to 'persuade' another coordinator to transfer a research subject to her industry-sponsored trial with the promise of a lucrative finder's fee. Residents have also been paid to recruit patients into clinical trials. CROs, for their part, enlist both academic and community-based physicians in the recruitment of subjects.[37] They generally emphasize their success in recruitment in marketing their services to pharmaceuticals corporations.[38] In response to the hunger for research subjects, companies have appeared specializing solely in patient recruitment.[39]

In some areas of specialization (e.g., cardiology and psychiatry), where highly profitable drugs have spurred great interest from pharmaceuticals companies, the problem of access to research subjects has been made worse by the fierce competition. Corporate sponsors feel pressured to offer all available incentives to encourage recruitment of subjects for research in these areas. The extent of the pressure is evident in reports of recruitment firms using young female employees, offered bonuses running in the thousands of dollars, to recruit largely male schizophrenic patients.[40]

Ethical Issues: Finder's Fees – Threatening Therapeutic Obligations?

The principal concern with finder's fees is that they may unduly influence the judgment of physicians as to the appropriateness of research participation for their patients. Finder's fees, in other words, give rise to a conflict between physicians' financial interests in patient recruitment, and their patients' interests in receiving their physicians' unbiased judgment as to what is in their best medical interests. When the research involves healthy subjects, the conflict is one between physicians' personal financial interests and their obligation to protect the prospective subjects from harm.

Financial interests may drive physicians to behave differently when recruiting patients or volunteers for clinical trials.[41] The influence of financial interests may become manifest in a number of ways, many of which might not be readily perceptible. Researchers in a position of conflict might become more lenient with respect to informed consent procedures, they may convince themselves that research participation is in their patient's best interests, or they may be overly flexible with regard to the study inclusion and exclusion criteria.[42] As mentioned earlier, several reports indicate that the lure of financial gain has in the recent past compromised the judgment of some health care professionals in these ways.[43] At a 2000 NIH conference on conflict of interest, Dr Thomas Bodenheimer testified that financial pressures lead physicians to 'stretch the inclusion and exclusion criteria to enroll as many patients as they can, thereby compromising the trial's validity. Physicians have been reported to enroll patients who do not even have the disease being studied, and physicians with no knowledge of a disease being studied are participating in trials.'[44] The Office of Inspector General cites a sponsor representative who confirms this, reporting that some investigators use "'outrageously bad clinical judgement" just to get subjects into a trial.'[45]

Finder's fees give rise to another set of concerns, often overlooked and best understood within the wider context of the increasing commercial pressures on physicians involved in research. When financial interests in patient recruitment are significant, physicians may give priority to this type of activity over patient care. Particularly when access to care is scarce and waiting lists are significant, finder's fees can greatly exacerbate access issues, overburdening those physicians who have chosen not to spend a large proportion of their time recruiting patients and filling out forms against considerable payment. This phenomenon raises justice concerns, both insofar as the financial interests hamper patient access to care, and insofar as the burdens of providing that care may become unequally distributed among members of the profession. Although this issue may be more acute in the United States, where participation in research may sometimes be an easy way for the uninsured to have affordable access to health care, it is troubling also in Canada, where waiting lists for physicians in research-intensive specialties are often considerable. The large number of clinical trials for diseases affecting the elderly (major consumers of pharmaceuticals) may negatively affect access to geriatric care.[46] An increasing number of those involved in care for the elderly spend an increasing proportion of their time in clinical trials, thereby diverting resources from patient care. Governments and professional organizations should look into this issue, since it raises important questions concerning allocation of resources and the provision of essential medical services.

Increased waiting lists may, furthermore, compromise the informed consent process. When waiting lists for treatment are long, the prospect of participation in research often becomes a tempting route to care for anxious patients. Physicians involved in remunerative recruitment may be tempted to suggest to patients that research participation will give them faster access to care. In such circumstances, one of the core principles of research ethics is compromised – namely, that which requires research subjects' consent to participation to be free from undue influence or coercion. Patients' freedom of choice is affected where they are confronted with the choice of immediate treatment through research participation or delayed treatment through the normal routes of clinical care. How often this happens is hard to say. One of us has received personal testimony from a patient who was offered faster access to care through participation in a placebo-controlled trial for a new anti-depressant. This offer was made with explicit reference to the several month waiting list for psychotherapy, the treatment preferred by the patient.

Another problem created by finder's fees and other incentives relates to the quality of the research being conducted. Interviewed for the *Lancet*, Dr Richard A. Friedman stated that such incentives have created in the United States 'a whole industry of private physicians who don't necessarily have any experience in research or with protocols in the speciality areas in which they're testing.'[47] These physicians are most likely to participate as patient recruiters and data collectors, and less likely to be critically involved in the development of the study and analysis of the data. Others have pointed out that industry-sponsored clinical research is often characterized by careful selection of interventions and trial design.[48] Insofar as private physicians are often inexperienced in research, they are not in a position to assess the methods and objectives of study sponsors critically.

Furthermore, for both academic and non-academic researchers, data may be analysed by employees of the research sponsor, and the results discussed and written (or withheld, when detrimental to the sponsor) by company researchers.[49] There is indication that in some instances, companies determine the authorship of the prepared study results on the basis of physicians' patient enrolment figures.[50] The Office of Inspector General cites the following stipulation of a sponsor-investigator contract: 'The order on the author list will be determined by the number of patients enrolled, so that the centre which enrolls the highest number of patients will obtain first authorship.'[51]

These developments raise a host of issues. First, they mean that patients may be put at risk by participating in trials run by less qualified researchers, having been referred by physicians unfamiliar with the research. Second, the physicians involved in the research may be less committed or accustomed to following rigorous scientific processes. When the quality of research declines, so does the reliability of the outcome. Flaws in the way data are gathered may affect the reliability of the approval system for new drugs. Third, even when experienced researchers are involved, the lack of control over data analysis raises serious issues with respect to real or perceived bias. Fourth, and finally, problems such as these may be difficult to detect, given that authorship of the study will often be attributed to non-industry researchers, many of whom will be reputable.

The shift to community-based research makes it more important than ever to expose and address the weaknesses of our current research review systems. Community-based researchers often do not have access to institutional IRB/REBs, and therefore have to rely on IRB/REBs set up by and located within CROs, or alternatively on private commercial review boards. As we will discuss further below, these boards are in a structural conflict of interest, since they depend on contracts offered by clients who have a significant financial interest in seeing their research protocols approved. Moreover, some forms of private research may not be covered by existing research regulations or guidelines. In Canada, for example, the *Tri-Council Policy Statement* issued by the federal funding agencies is not uniformly enforceable. Health Canada's Therapeutic Products Directorate has declared that trials intended to lead to a drug approval application must abide by the statement. But it is not clear how this declaration would be enforced, and there is conflict between some of Health Canada's expectations related to clinical trials design and the requirements of the *Tri-Council Policy Statement* (e.g., those relating to placebo-controlled trials).

One traditionally expects commitment to independent research, intense scrutiny of trial design, and demanding interpretation of results from researchers within academic environments. Unfortunately, it has become evident that the need for private funding has rendered academic researchers increasingly vulnerable to conflicts of interest. The increased competition between community-based researchers and academic institutions may have the effect of undermining further the power of academic investigators to question and challenge protocols submitted by sponsors, and to push for publication of critical results. Several high-profile cases indicate that the financial interests of sponsors can lead them to interfere with the dissemination of results that are potentially commercially damaging.[52] As academic research institutions become increasingly dependent on industry-sponsored research, pressures to give priority to these trials over publicly funded investigator-driven research can be expected to increase.[53] Moreover, the comparatively low levels of funding may make it much harder to recruit patients for publicly funded research. It should be expected that as financial rewards continue to be offered as incentives to recruitment activity, other interests will suffer. The lure of finder's fees threatens more than physicians' fidelity to therapeutic obligations, patient access to care, and the consent process. It stands also to threaten the integrity of the scientific process, and to undermine public trust in science as a cooperative pursuit of basic social goods.[54]

IRB/REB Review of Finder's Fees and Conflicts of Interest

Conflict of interest has usefully been defined as 'a discrepancy between the personal interests and the professional responsibilities of a person in a position of trust.'[55] This definition highlights both moral and legal characteristics of the physician-patient relationship, importing notions of professional responsibility and fiduciary duty. From our discussion to this point, it should be evident that finder's fees risk adding significantly to existing conflicts of interest in research – an enterprise already characterized by fundamental tension between the ends of research and clinical care. A number of existing mechanisms can be employed to analyse and mediate conflicts of interest.

As has been highlighted by various commentators, IRB/REBs can play a significant role in assessing the potential impact of conflicts of interest on research.[56] In the United States, existing federal regulations governing human subjects research fail specifically to instruct IRBs to assess conflicts of interest.[57] The FDA has specified in its *Information Sheets* that IRBs should review the methods and materials investigators will use to recruit patients,[58] but there is no requirement that investigators disclose payments or other incentives related to recruitment activity. It is therefore not surprising that the Office of Inspector General found that 75 per cent of U.S. IRBs they surveyed 'do not review any financial arrangements between sponsors and investigators.'[59] More remarkable is that 'few inquire about specific recruitment practices.'[60]

The Department of Health and Human Services (DHHS) and the FDA both introduced in the 1990s regulations regarding the disclosure of the financial conflicts of interest of clinical investigators.[61] The DHHS regulations oblige federally funded institutions to obtain annual financial disclosure statements from investigators who participate in funded research, and to evaluate whether their financial interests in research are such as to possibly affect the conduct of research. The FDA regulations are directed towards research intended to lead to application for the approval of a drug or medical device. They oblige sponsors of such research to collect information on financial interests and to disclose this information when submitting the results of the study. While both sets of regulations have increased awareness of many important

issues and promoted the development of conflict of interest committees in many institutions, they are nevertheless insufficient.[62] They do
not clearly prohibit certain forms of conflict of interest, nor do they
provide a clear mandate or adequate guidance to IRBs as to appropriate measures for responding to conflicts of interest.

There is pressure to close this gap in the regulatory mandate of IRBs.
Under the direction of Donna Shalala, former secretary of health and
human services, the DHHS showed signs of movement in the direction
of improving regulatory control of conflict of interest. She promised
that her department would introduce regulations, develop new guidelines, and encourage legislation providing civil penalties for violations
of ethics requirements, ranging up to $250,000 for investigators, and
$1 million for institutions.[63] The DHHS has developed a final guid-
ance document on conflicts of interest in which it recognizes the need
for thorough IRB review of financial interests of both investigators and
institutions, as well as consideration of any financial conflicts of interest by the institutions themselves.[64] The final guidance document
acknowledges that conflicts of interest may compromise the rights and
welfare of research subjects. It accordingly recommends that IRBs, as
well as institutions and investigators, obtain information about these
interests and carefully scrutinize them in the review process and provides guidance on how to remove or minimize any conflicts of interest
found. The final guidance document fails, however, to clearly delineate
limits on conflicts of interest. It is uncertain whether such limits may be
established through the promulgation of specific regulations in the
future, as it is unclear whether the commitment expressed by Donna
Shalala is shared by current secretary Tommy G. Thompson. In this
respect, the controversy over the membership of the newly created
Secretary's Advisory Committee on Human Research Protections
(SACHRP) raises concerns. Most members represent institutions or
organizations with financial interests in research.[65]

Other initiatives appear more promising, although lacking in regulatory force and limited in scope to academic institutions. A special task
force of the Association of American Medical Colleges has made relevant recommendations in two reports, one on institutional conflicts of
interest, the other on conflicts of interest suffered by investigators.[66]
The task force recommends, among other things, that institutions
develop policies that impose a rebuttable presumption that investigators' significant financial interest in research bars their participation. It
also acknowledges that various forms of financial relations – including

membership on advisory boards and paid speaking engagements – generate conflicts of interest. It further recommends that IRBs be fully informed of financial interests and evaluate their potential impact on proposed research. The task force goes so far as to suggest that institutions not permit research to be conducted in their own institution where conflicts of interest are significant. Again, no clear prohibitions are introduced, but at least there is an acknowledgment of the need for thorough review.

With respect to the assessment of conflicts of interests in the research review process, the situation in Canada seems, at least prima facie, to compare favourably with that of the United States. It is therefore worth discussing in more detail. In Canada, REBs are charged with considerable responsibility when it comes to assessing conflicts of interest, as part of their overall mandate to protect human research subjects. Health Canada's Therapeutic Products Directorate (TPD) confirms in an Impact Analysis Statement accompanying new regulations on clinical trials that REBs help to 'ensure that conflict of interest situations are avoided and that the health and safety of the trial subjects remain the paramount concern.'[67] However, while the regulations recognize the increasingly important role of REBs, they do not provide a regulatory framework for REB review or for the oversight of REBs.

The *Tri-Council Policy Statement* specifies several types of conflicts of interest to be addressed by REBs. It is issued by Canada's major federal research funding agencies, but has been explicitly recognized by the TPD as expressing core ethical standards for research related to the drug approval process. The funding agencies are entering into contractual agreements with funded institutions.[68] These contracts stipulate that the institutions will respect the *Tri-Council Policy Statement* for all of their research. Through its incorporation as a contractual term, the reach of the statement exceeds the bounds of agency-funded research.

Article 4.1 of the *Tri-Council Policy Statement* requires researchers and others involved in the research to disclose 'actual, perceived or potential conflicts of interest to the REB.' Where the REB has reason to believe conflicts have not been disclosed, or have been disclosed inadequately, it has the power to withhold approval pending adequate disclosure. In discharging its duty to identify and assess the nature and degree of reported conflicts, REBs may access and scrutinize 'details of the research project, budgets, commercial interests, consultative relationships and other relevant information.'[69] Again, if the REB has reason to believe that such material information is being withheld, it would be within its authority to suspend approval pending compliance with its demands. While REBs may not have the authority directly to halt ongoing research, they could report any deficiencies to the appropriate federal, provincial, and agency authorities.

REBs are further required to ensure that payments to investigators per participant are not disproportionate to standard professional fees.[70] However, REBs may have great difficulty in identifying conflicts owing to disproportionate fees, given that the fees are often well hidden within the budgets of research projects. Demanding access to the relevant information (in this case, the budget) may not help REBs to identify and assess the extent of the conflict. Moreover, it is unclear whether REBs currently analyse budgets of clinical trials appropriately or receive detailed information on these trials by contract officers within their institutions.

REBs are additionally expected to address conflicts of interest that may influence the informed consent process. For consent to be fully informed, and thus adequate, research subjects must be apprised of all information that could reasonably be expected to be material to their decision whether to participate. Clearly, it is only reasonable to expect that information relating to the financial interests of the researchers and referring physicians in the research would be material to this decision. The *Tri-Council Policy Statement* recognizes this in part by requiring REBs to ensure that consent documents disclose 'the presence of any ... conflict of interest on the part of researchers, their institutions or sponsors.'[71] Considering the wide range of possible sources of conflict and the ways in which they may be hidden, we suggest that this requirement also presents a daunting challenge for REBs. In order fully to appraise the adequacy of proposed disclosure of financial interests, REBs must have a complete profile detailing in plain terms the financial relations between referring physicians, the researchers, and the sponsors. Speaking engagements, contracts for expert consultant work, personal investments, and so on, ought to be included in such profiles. It seems unlikely that REBs would currently be capable of obtaining such information, let alone assessing it. Regulatory agencies, universities, and research institutes ought to assist REBs in this respect by creating more demanding disclosure obligations and developing channels of communication between contract offices and REBs. Employment contracts should specify disclosure as a contractual obligation.

Given the existence of research ethics review, the detailed requirements for research ethics approval, and the seemingly significant powers of the REBs, it would seem reasonable in the Canadian context to assume that subjects will be adequately protected from the negative effects of conflicts of interest by REBs. Canadian physicians referring their patients to research might avoid investigating adequately whether participation would be in their best medical interests, or whether their fees should be a source of concern, comforted by their awareness of the relevant provisions of the *Tri-Council Policy Statement* and their expectation that these can and will be enforced as a matter of routine by REBs.

While REBs are fulfilling an increasingly important role in overseeing research, significant and serious weaknesses in the Canadian research review system, coupled with the lack of regulatory oversight, make it inappropriate for Canadian authorities to treat REB review as an adequate control mechanism.[72] Researchers, sponsors, funding agencies, and academic institutions should be aware that the courts are unlikely to find that REB approval relieves them from their legal obligations to research subjects.[73]

A number of problems ought to be kept in mind. Many REBs across Canada and IRBs in the United States find themselves overburdened with review and related administrative responsibilities.[74] In high-volume research centres, review boards often simply lack the time to carry out the rigorous and thorough review required to ensure that the conditions discussed above are upheld. We further suspect that most boards do not have the expertise required for detailed analysis of budgets. Given that finder's fees may be hidden in study budgets (i.e., allocated across a number of different categories of expenses), in order to identify and assess budgets for the presence of finder's fees, review boards would need to have a fairly sophisticated sense of what constitutes reasonable research expenses by category.

In addition to time- and resource-related problems are more systemic considerations. Although REBs are increasingly recognized as crucial administrative entities,[75] they remain remarkably under-regulated. As pointed out earlier, new Canadian clinical trials regulations rely on REBs to assess conflicts of interest and to ensure that research subjects are adequately protected, but in the Impact Analysis Statement accompanying the regulations it is admitted that 'REBs that review and approve the conduct of human clinical trials in Canada are not currently subject to federal regulations or accreditation,' and that 'some REBs have limited resources and experience with the review of drug clinical trials.'[76] Neither the funding agencies' *Tri-Council Policy*

Statement nor the *ICH Good Clinical Practice* (*ICH GCP*) guideline, introduced by cross-reference as the regulatory framework by the TPD, enjoys the status of law. They are guidelines, and while their dictates are in certain cases made binding through contract, they cannot thereby be extended to all forms of research. Furthermore, while Canadian funding agencies, the Canadian National Council on Ethics in Human Research, and Health Canada's Ethics Division are currently looking into developing standards for the accreditation of REBs and certification of REB members, there is currently no system for sustained and thorough oversight of REBs.[77] Preliminary review of compliance with the federal funding agencies' guidelines has started, but is still in its early stages. Given this, it is not surprising, although no less disturbing, that several REBs in Canada have allegedly approved with impunity clinical trials protocols that clearly violate one of the provisions of the *Tri-Council Policy Statement*.[78] Although the requirement breached has been the subject of considerable debate,[79] it is clearly inimical to the integrity of the system that the bodies charged with oversight be permitted to disregard the substantive conditions they are obliged to enforce without immediate intervention by regulatory and funding agencies.

It is clear that while REBs are expected to enforce the requirements of the *Tri-Council Policy Statement* or the *ICH GCP* guideline, they are not made accountable for their failure to do so. The TPD requires sponsors of clinical trials to submit a 'Research Ethics Board Attestation' with their request to conduct a clinical trial involving a new investigational drug. This attestation must be signed by the chair of an REB and kept on file by the trial sponsor for twenty-five years. Aside from identifying information on the REB and its chair, no further information about the REB or its review is required. REBs can be established without abiding by any specific procedural requirements (regarding the selection of members, for example), without going through any formal approval process, and they conduct their business without ongoing oversight. REBs have only to declare in the above-mentioned attestations that they are constituted and function in accordance with the *Tri-Council Policy Statement* and the *ICH GCP* guideline. As a result, REBs across Canada differ markedly in terms of the number of their members, the constitution of their membership, and their relationship to researchers and research sponsors. Although more formal regulation is present in the United States, similar problems of oversight of IRBs have been highlighted in several reports and in the literature.[80]

In the United States and in Canada, IRB/REBs operate traditionally within academic institutions, and are comprised of members drawn from a range of disciplines and scientific specialties within the institution. That said, the demand for, and number of, commercial review boards is growing. Several specialized for-profit commercial boards have been set up in North America, reviewing research protocols against payment of considerable review fees. These boards are particularly important for the review of the community-based clinical trials in which finder's fees are prominent. Community-based researchers often do not have access to academic review boards, and commercial for-profit boards offer their services to fill this gap. Several CROs have also set up inhouse boards, which attract external members through payment of consultant's fees. With the rise of for-profit and inhouse review boards, review has itself become invested in the lucrative research industry. Many of these boards may be diligent in performing their reviews;[81] however, as has been discussed elsewhere, it seems extraordinary and highly inappropriate that review boards with a vested interest in the success of their clients are relied upon blindly to serve the public interest in protecting research subjects and controlling conflicts of interest.[82] In consideration of the enormous pressures on recruitment, inhouse boards seem that much more problematic. If speedy recruitment is crucial to the economic fortunes of research sponsors, is it wise public policy to rely on inhouse review boards to identify and prohibit inappropriate recruitment incentives?

The rise of for-profit and inhouse review boards means that already significant problems associated with the lack of oversight and uniform standards for research review are exacerbated by another: the possibility that corporate sponsors may engage in forum shopping.[83] Even if most such boards are scrupulous in their enforcement of conflict of interest provisions, one lenient board can create considerable havoc. Nothing currently prevents sponsors or researchers from establishing their own review boards, or shopping for more lenient boards when a study is rejected by the board of an academic institution. Moreover, sponsor-friendly commercial boards can be established and dissolved very quickly, thereby potentially escaping legal liability. One private ethics committee embroiled in a controversy relating to the approval of a study involving the importation of poor research subjects into Switzerland indicated in its Internet advertisements that it could set up in different countries 'on request.'[84]

This is not to suggest that academic and other institutional review boards do not suffer from important conflict of interest issues. Conflicts of interest are also a problem in institutional boards, where members are often reviewing protocols submitted by close colleagues or superiors.[85] Furthermore, the increasing financial interest, even outright dependence, of some academic institutions on lucrative commercial research erodes the distinction between academic and inhouse boards.[86] Members of academic review boards may sometimes themselves feel the financial pressures facing their institution, as for example where they realize what the rejection of a lucrative study could mean for funding of research at the institution.[87] While some of these conflicts are inherent in institutional review systems, and may often be compensated for by the integrity and commitment of dedicated members, others reflect fundamental shifts in research funding, as academic institutions in an era of government fiscal restraint look to corporate sponsorship as an important source of revenue. The very environment that makes IRB/REB review ever more important threatens the integrity of the system as it currently functions. The pressures generated by this environment on researchers, review boards, and host institutions give further indication of the need for restructuring and regulatory consolidation of the research ethics review system.

Discussion of precisely how the research review system ought to be reformed is beyond the scope of this paper. It must suffice here to note that other jurisdictions have, in our view, better recognized the significant public policy mandate served by review boards.[88] Given that they are mandated to protect the rights and welfare of research subjects, the boards ought to be given a sound administrative structure, akin to those enjoyed by other quasi-judicial administrative bodies, and developed with a view to protecting their independence. It is worth noting in connection with the earlier mentioned VanTx scandal that a Swiss Bundesgericht recently confirmed in an appeal decision that the cantonal authorities have the authority to assign exclusive authority to a regional research review board, thereby depriving private review boards within their jurisdiction of their authority to operate. The board involved in this scandal had challenged a 2000 decision by the cantonal government of Basel to give exclusive research review authority to one regional board. The highest court ruled that the organization of research review is part of the cantons' legitimate exercise of state authority in matters of health protection. Although it did not rule out that private parties could play a role in this system, it explicitly stated that they could only do so under explicit delegation of authority from the health authorities. 'A research ethics committee fulfills a control function with a mandate from the state,' the court ruled, 'and the exercise of such function should not be open to whoever is interested.'[89]

A similar statement recognizing the administrative mandate of IRBs and the concomitant importance of full independence was made in the recent controversial decision of the Maryland Court of Appeal in *Grimes v. Kennedy Krieger Institute*. The court in *Grimes* suggested that institutional IRBs might lack the independence requisite to their fulfilling adequately their important mandate.[90]

The Ethical and Legal Responsibilities of Physicians Involved in Research: Professional Guidelines

At least until decent national regulatory structures are implemented and meaningful oversight and enforcement is provided for, it should not simply be assumed that research subjects will be adequately protected from unacceptable risks and the influence of untoward conflicts by IRB/REBs. Physicians and others involved in research should question the appropriateness of their financial interests in research and, at a minimum, should disclose them to institutional authorities and research subjects.

There are also legal reasons for researchers to avoid mere reliance upon IRB/REB review. As Bernard Dickens observes, 'a lapse of due care by ... [a] Research Ethics Board may not exonerate the investigator, but rather afford a research subject remedies against the REB institution, for negligence or, for instance, breach of fiduciary duty.'[91] The physicians and other health professionals involved in research have the best opportunity, and an independent obligation, to determine whether research participation is in the best interests of their patients. In meeting that obligation, they must avoid even the appearance of conflict, in recognition of the fact that fiduciary relationships are relationships of trust that 'can be put at risk by conflicts of interest that may compromise independence, objectivity or ethical duties of loyalty.'[92] Researchers, physicians, and others involved in research are obliged to familiarize themselves with research ethics guidelines and to treat these as binding professional standards governing their personal involvement in all research-related activities.

The existence of an independent obligation bearing on the conduct of individual physicians in industry-sponsored research is recognized in both Canadian and American professional ethics guidelines. The

Canadian Medical Association's (CMA) policy statement, *Physicians and the Pharmaceutical Industry*,[93] adopts the following as a guiding principle: 'The practising physician's primary obligation is to the patient. Relationships with industry are appropriate only insofar as they do not negatively affect the fiduciary nature of the patient-physician relationship.'[94] The CMA policy expressly treats finder's fees as follows:

> It is acceptable for physicians to receive remuneration for enrolling patients or participating in approved research studies only if such activity exceeds their normal practice pattern. This remuneration should not constitute enticement. It may, however, replace income lost as a result of participating in a study. Parameters such as time expenditure and complexity of the study may also be relevant considerations. The amount of the remuneration should be approved by the relevant review board, agency or body ... Research subjects must be informed if their physician will receive a fee for enrolling them in a study.[95]

While the CMA statement seems intended to dissuade researchers from accepting finder's fees, and while it does call attention to the independent obligations of physicians with respect to their treatment of patients and management of conflicts, it is not without its problems. First and foremost, it does not clearly and unequivocally prohibit finder's fees (i.e., fees that cannot reasonably be said to be proportionate to services provided). Indeed, it exceeds normal practice patterns to spend five minutes talking to patients about a clinical trial or to call up a sponsor's agent. Is it appropriate for physicians to receive financial reward for short phone conversations?

Additionally, the CMA statement fails to provide clear guidance on how much time physicians should be devoting to patient recruitment activities when demands for clinical care are high. Further, while it provides that fees should be disclosed, it does not mention that significant fees may be hidden in study budgets. It should state that physicians are to be attuned to such hidden fees and that they are responsible for disclosing them. Finally, the CMA policy mentions that finder's fees should be disclosed to patients, but it does not clearly indicate that the amount of the fees should be disclosed. We would argue that the quantum of fees must be disclosed to subjects, for otherwise they have no way of distinguishing between the physician who receives fees commensurate with standard professional fees, and the physician whose fees are excessive and perhaps a source of undue influence. Finally, the guidelines could recognize the other ways in which financial interests affect recruitment practices, and detail physicians' responsibilities with regard to these.

By contrast, the guidance of the American Medical Association (AMA) is spare, but clear and unequivocal. The AMA prohibits finder's fees without exception. The Council on Ethical and Judicial Affairs of the AMA addresses the issues underlying finder's fees in a general statement on conflicts of interest in research, and in a separate opinion makes a direct statement on finder's fees.

In its opinion, *Conflicts of Interest: Biomedical Research*, the council stresses that the 'avoidance of real or perceived conflicts of interest in clinical research is imperative' to ensuring the maintenance of trust in the integrity of both institutions and individuals members the medical community.[96] On this basis, it recommends that institutions adopt a series of rules on conflicts of interest, one of which is of particular relevance. This rule requires that 'any remuneration received by the researcher from the company whose product is being studied ... be commensurate with the efforts of the researcher on behalf of the company.'[97]

Perhaps recognizing that the implications of this recommendation for finder's fees are not straightforward, the AMA council issued a statement on finder's fees in their opinion, *Fee Splitting: Referrals to Health Care Facilities*.[98] In this opinion, the council states simply, and without elaboration, that 'offering or accepting payment for referring patients to research studies (finder's fees) is unethical.'[99] This statement does not distinguish legitimate recovery of administrative expenses from finder's fees, nor does it acknowledge the difficulty of making this distinction in practice, but it seems reasonable to infer that what is prohibited is the offer and acceptance of fees for the act of referral per se, over and above recovery of actual costs. This inference is reasonable if the opinion on finder's fees is to be read in conjunction with the earlier statement calling for commensurability between remuneration and services provided. Additionally, it is interesting to note that the AMA prohibition targets not only physicians who may be enticed by offers of finder's fees, but also those who would offer them.

Subsequent to issuing its opinion on finder's fees, the AMA council received several requests for clarification. It responded to these requests in its report, *Finder's Fees: Payment for the Referral of Patients to Clinical Research Studies*.[100] Essentially, the council reiterates much of the earlier opinion, elaborating slightly in declaring that: 'it is unethical for physicians to receive any kind of compensation in return for the referral of patients to health care facilities. By prohibiting referral fees paid to physicians by "clinics, laboratories, hospitals or other health care facilities," the opinion covers referral fees for research studies as well, since such studies must be conducted in a health care facility.'[101] This clarification of the AMA position is interesting in at least three ways. First, the issue of finder's fees in research is set in the context of a position on the ethicality of referral fees in clinical contexts more broadly. It thus affirms the primary importance of the physician's obligation to act in the best interests of his or her patient in making all manner of referrals. Second, and significantly, there is an expanded sense of what may be included under the rubric of 'finder's fees.' Any kind of compensation will count; it is not only fees per se that are prohibited. Third, and finally, the prohibition on offering finder's fees is no longer explicitly mentioned. It seems logical, however, to presume that this practice remains frowned upon by the council. If the council condemns the behaviour of physicians who accept finder's fees, it should have the same opinion of physicians offering them. The fact that offering fees is no longer mentioned points perhaps to the fact that fees are most often offered by trial sponsors who are not physicians and over whom the council feels it has no moral authority.

In sum, while the CMA policy on finder's fees is well intentioned, its position is not clear and unequivocal on its face, nor is the guidance provided adequate. The AMA statement has its shortcomings (for example, more could have been said to assist physicians in identifying finder's fees, and in explanation of the basis for the prohibition), but we feel its clear prohibition on finder's fees is both justified and preferable to the qualified, noncommittal content and tenor of the CMA policy.

The policies developed by medical associations obviously do not have the status of law, but they do define standards for professional conduct. They should be publicized more widely and enforced to the extent possible by the CMA and AMA. Greater awareness of the problems associated with finder's fees could be generated through educational sessions at annual meetings, or through collaboration with medical schools on the development of specific educational programs for medical students.

Legal Remedies

More powerful mechanisms for enforcing the obligations of physicians involved in research are found in statutory and common law. Physicians involved in research have strict obligations to patients under law, but they may often be unaware of the way in which these obligations constrain their relationships with industry. There are both statutory and common law grounds upon which a legal complaint involving finder's fees could be brought against the physicians receiving the fee and possibly the host institutions.

To begin with, it should be noted that in the United States, finder's fees may attract prosecution under the federal *False Claims Act*[102] and the *Anti-Kickback Statute.*[103] The various ways these statutes can be applied to counter unethical practices in research have been highlighted and discussed in detail in an important article by Paul E. Kalb and Kristin G. Koehler.[104] They argue that researchers and host institutions could be charged by federal authorities under the *False Claims Act* for fraud in their submission of claims for reimbursement of research expenses to federal funding agencies (the *False Claims Act* 'prohibits the "knowing" submission of false or fraudulent claims and false statements to the government').[105] The *False Claims Act* could thus be applied in prosecution of researchers and institutions who claim reimbursement of finder's fees by hiding the costs associated with providing them within other budgetary categories. To avoid prosecution, researchers and institutions must disclose in a clear and complete manner all expenses related to the recruitment of research subjects. Kalb and Koehler note that the *False Claims Act* could also be applied in prosecution of institutions and individual researchers for failure to comply with federal regulations requiring written assurance of compliance.[106] This would encompass failures to comply with the Common Rule[107] and FDA human subjects regulations,[108] as well as those requiring institutional assessment of conflicts of interest and disclosure of same to federal authorities.[109] Finally, Kalb and Koehler draw attention to the fact that the *Anti-Kickback Statute* makes it a felony for manufacturers and clinicians to make payments intended to induce referral of patients covered by federal health programs including Medicare and Medicaid.[110] This would include inducement through payment of finder's fees for referrals of patients to trials funded in part by federal health programs. Significant penalties are attached to violations of both the *False Claims Act* and the *Anti-Kickback Statute*. Individual researchers and institutions could face fines under the *False Claims Act* ranging from tens of thousands to tens of millions of dollars.[111] The felony offence under the *Anti-Kickback Statute* provides for severe fines and imprisonment for up to five years on conviction.[112]

Rules about kickbacks in medical practice also exist in all but two Canadian provinces. The mechanisms to deal with kickbacks vary greatly from province to province in terms of the type of legal instrument and the scope of relevant provisions. They are either regulated through by-laws of colleges of physicians and surgeons, or through statutes and regulations governing the medical profession.[113] Finder's fees would likely be deemed to amount to kickbacks for referrals.

In Ontario, a statutory basis for conflict-of-interest related complaints is found in the *Medicine Act*.[114] The *Medicine Act* sets out a number of provisions that provide the basis for determinations of professional misconduct for the purposes of section 51(1)(c) of the *Health Professions Procedural Code*.[115] The *Medicine Act* is enforced by the Discipline Committee of the College of Physicians and Surgeons of Ontario. Several of the provisions of the *Medicine Act* may provide a basis for bringing charges of professional misconduct against physicians who accept finder's fees or who have a financial interest in research to which they refer their patients. Section 1(1)(5), provides, for example, that 'having a conflict of interest' is an act of professional misconduct. Conflict of interest is defined in the *Medicine Act* as follows:

> 17. (1) It is a conflict of interest for a member to order a diagnostic or therapeutic service to be performed by a facility in which the member or a member of his or her family has a proprietary interest unless ... (a) the fact of the proprietary interest is disclosed to the patient before a service is performed ...[116]

It could be argued that physicians who refer patients to a clinical trial in which they have a financial interest are 'ordering a diagnostic or therapeutic service' from a 'facility' in which they have a financial interest. While section 1(1)(5) of the *Medicine Act* ought to catch many of the circumstances in which finder's fees are accepted, its application seems limited in at least two ways by the definition. First, it is unclear whether all research for which finder's fees are accepted could be considered 'a diagnostic or therapeutic service.' It is unlikely that this could be said to be the case for research involving healthy volunteers, for example. Second, it is unclear whether there could be a charge of professional misconduct for conflict of interest if the research was not performed in a facility owned or operated by the sponsor offering the fee. We would argue that the financial interest of the referring physician should be understood as following the research no matter where it is conducted. It is worth pointing out that several physicians have established independent administrative entities for the conduct of clinical trials. If they refer their patients to these 'facilities' in order to enrol them in a clinical trial, they clearly refer them to a facility in which they have a financial interest.

In circumstances to which section 1(1)(5) applies, it appears that disclosure of the conflict relieves the physician from a charge of professional misconduct. That said, a charge could be brought where there were flaws in the quality and manner of disclosure. Since the legal standard of disclosure for research is that of complete and detailed disclosure, research subjects must be informed in reasonable detail of every potential conflict. Full and frank disclosure means that physicians are obliged to disclose the quantum of the fee received per referral, even if these payments would be used to fund other research projects. Furthermore, it also crucial that other financial relations between the sponsor, researcher, and referring physician be disclosed, since these may also influence those involved in the recruitment process. For that reason, researchers should disclose paid speaking obligations, consulting relations, personal investments, and so on.

Section 1(1)(11) of the *Medicine Act* prohibits '[s]haring fees with a person who has referred a patient or receiving fees from any person to whom a member has referred a patient.' Section 1(1)(21) makes it professional misconduct to '[c]harge a fee that is excessive in relation to services performed.' Although both provisions are clearly aimed at clinical practice contexts, nothing seems to bar one from invoking them in the context of research. The first provision could make it an offence to receive from another physician money merely for referral of patients to a clinical trial. The second could apply when an excessive fee is charged merely for the referral of a subject to a clinical trial.

Another interesting provision is section 1(1)(10) of the *Medicine Act*, which makes it an act of professional misconduct to give information concerning the condition of a patient to a third party without the patient's consent. The requirement of consent should be kept in mind in institutions where physicians receive fees for bringing 'interesting' potential subjects to the attention of their colleagues.

Finally, section 1(1)(33) provides that a physician may be charged with professional misconduct for 'an act or omission relevant to the practice of medicine that, having regard to all the circumstances, would reasonably be regarded by members as disgraceful, dishonourable or unprofessional.' This provision ought to capture truly egregious situations, such as the acceptance of excessive fees, harassment of patients for their participation or misrepresentation aimed at inducing patients to participate, the acceptance of fees for referral of patients to research of questionable scientific quality, referrals to trials that expose patients to significant and unnecessary risk, and participation in such trials. There are even stronger legal mechanisms available. Physicians involved in remunerated recruitment activity ought to be aware of their legal obligations as defined by the courts.[117] If a court finds that a physician has failed entirely, or adequately, to inform his or her patient of information relevant to the patient's decision whether to participate, the physician could be held liable in tort for battery or negligence (depending on whether fraud or misrepresentation is involved).[118] The Supreme Court of Canada, in *Reibl v. Hughes*[119] and *Hopp v. Lepp*,[120] has held that physicians must disclose all information that would be deemed material by a reasonable person in the circumstances of their patients, to the extent that these circumstances ought to be known to the physician. Ellen Picard and Gerald Robertson speculate on the basis of existing case law that 'a Canadian court would impose a duty on the doctor to inform the patient of the conflict of interest.'[121] They surmise that 'the possibility that an interest extraneous to the patient's health has affected the physician's judgement is something that a reasonable patient would want to know ... It is material to the patient's decision and, thus, a prerequisite to informed consent.'[122] The emphasis on full disclosure follows from the courts' interpretation of the nature of the physician-patient relationship. Fiduciary relations impose higher standards of full and frank exchange of important information.[123]

As confirmed in the leading Canadian case, *Halushka v. University of Saskatchewan*, the obligation to disclose information pertinent to patient consent is even more demanding in the context of research.[124] The court in *Halushka* concluded that '[t]he subject of medical experimentation is entitled to a full and frank disclosure of all the facts, probabilities and opinions which a reasonable man might be expected to consider before giving his consent.'[125] This was confirmed in *Weiss v. Solomon*, a case in which both the researcher and the institution whose REB had permitted the study were held liable for exposing a subject to risks of research without first obtaining appropriate consent.[126]

In the well-known U.S. case, *Moore v. Regents of the University of California*,[127] the legal ramifications of non-disclosure of the financial interests of a physician investigator was one of the core issues to be decided by the court. In *Moore*, the California Supreme Court delivered the strongest statement by a court yet of the obligation of physicians to disclose their personal interests in research to their patients. The court held that 'a physician must disclose personal interests unrelated to the patient's health, whether research or economic, that may affect the physician's professional judgment; and a physician's failure to disclose such interests may give rise to a cause of action for performing medical procedures without informed consent or breach of fiduciary duty.'[128] The court in *Moore* recognized a distinction between types of information to be disclosed – namely, between material risks and the physician's personal financial interests – but it held that the legal doctrine of informed consent 'is broad enough to encompass the latter.'[129]

Physicians involved in research should note that their common law obligations in situations of conflict of interest might extend beyond the duty of disclosure. It would be possible for a claim to be brought in which egregious finder's fees were cited as evidence of breach of fiduciary duty.[130]

Marc Rodwin describes the special characteristics of fiduciaries and fiduciary relationships as follows: 'Fiduciaries advise and represent others and manage their affairs. Usually they have specialized knowledge or expertise. Their work requires judgment and discretion. Often the party that the fiduciary serves cannot effectively monitor the fiduciary's performance. The fiduciary relationship is based on dependence, reliance and trust.'[131] These characteristics seem generally to aptly describe the power advantage enjoyed by physicians over their patients, particularly where their patients are ill.

The Supreme Court of Canada has shown interest in the law of fiduciary duty as a means to define the legal obligations of physicians to their patients. While the court was divided in the way it decided the case (in part as a result of the pleadings), the opinion of Justice McLachlin, as she then was, in *Norberg v. Wynrib* indicates that the court might recognize claims of breach of fiduciary duty as distinct from claims under tort or contract, in consideration of the power inequality characteristic of the physician-patient relationship.[132] McLachlin J. held that 'perhaps the most fundamental characteristic of the doctor-patient relationship is its fiduciary nature.'[133]

While the presence of consent may be sufficient for the purposes of tort and contract law – where parties are, in McLachlin J.'s words, 'taken to be independent and equal actors' – under the law of fiduciary duty, physicians may be held to a higher standard of conduct.[134] The judgment of McLachlin J. in *Norberg* stands as recognition of the legal significance of the fact that fiduciary relationships are characterized by 'the trust of a person with inferior power that another person who has assumed superior power and responsibility will exercise that power for his or her good and only for his or her good and in his or her best interests.'[135] If physicians compromise their therapeutic obligations to their patients because of the prospect of finder's fees, they violate their legally recognized obligation to 'act in the best interests' of their patients. McLachlin J. held that 'classic duties associated with a fiduciary relationship' include 'loyalty, good faith, and the avoidance of a conflict of duty and self-interest.'[136] In accepting finder's fees, physicians certainly put themselves in a position of conflict of duty and self-interest.

Ernest Weinrib has suggested that, given the nature of the wrong, the most appropriate remedy for breach of fiduciary duty is restitution of any gain realized through the breach.[137] This would mean a researcher found liable for breach of fiduciary duty would have to pay damages of an amount equal to the finder's fee. The courts have shown willingness to go further in awarding damages for breach of fiduciary duty. In *Norberg*, McLachlin J. indicated that the court's aim in such cases is to redress abuse of the balance of power enjoyed by the fiduciary, and that in doing so, it may be more generous in awarding remedies. In *Norberg*, this meant an award of punitive damages, in addition to the customary compensatory damages. The financial consequences of a finding of breach of fiduciary duty by Canadian courts may be increasingly significant. The Supreme Court of Canada recently sent a strong message to those engaging in what it considers 'misconduct that represents a marked departure from ordinary standards of decent behaviour' by upholding an unprecedented award of $1 million in punitive damages.[138]

It has been suggested that the legal significance of the fiduciary nature of the physician-patient relationship may be diminished by the increasing emphasis on the doctrine of informed consent. Bernard Dickens, for instance, suggests that 'courts may ... find less need to hold health care professionals to protective duties, and may place healthcare professional-patient relations among those of an arms length character in the nature of commerce between equals. The law's momentum toward patient empowerment may be on a collision course with judgments finding patients to be dependent and entitled to protection.'[139]

Similarly, in consideration of U.S. case law and its implications for understanding the legal obligations of physicians with regard to conflicts of interest, Marc Rodwin takes note of the fact that 'since the advent of informed consent litigation in the 1970s, patients have participated more in treatment decisions.'[140] Yet Rodwin sees this development as one best understood to be *within* the fiduciary conception of the patient-physician relationship. He acknowledges that 'informed consent promotes disclosure as part of a fiduciary ideal,' but warns of the importance of recognizing that even in an age of respect for the decision-making authority of patients, 'physicians still exercise significant power over patients' medical affairs. Patients [often] rely on physicians ... to exercise independent judgement and to make significant decisions for them.'[141] Particularly in light of the changes within the health care environment, we would hope that courts would continue to recognize that 'patients are usually in a poor position to monitor physicians, to second-guess their judgement, or to discover and sanction breaches of trust.'[142] As Fleetwood puts it, in connection with the disclosure of finder's fees, 'even if a conflict of interest is disclosed to the patient ... it would be tough for a patient to know what to do with, or how to respond to, the information. From the patient's perspective, physicians are always paid for their services, so why would enrolling a patient into a clinical trial be any different?'[143]

While commentators have seemed by and large reluctant to discuss common law remedies for conflicts of interest in research, the reluctance to entertain the applicability of criminal sanctions seems even more widespread. This seeming reluctance may merely be a reflection of the presumption that no Criminal Code provisions apply in conflict of interest situations. Picard and Robertson, for instance, have suggested that physicians' failure to inform patients of conflicts of interest will not trigger criminal sanctions.[144] We feel that this suggestion may merit reconsideration. While appeal to criminal sanctions may not be the most appropriate means through which to redress misconduct in research, if some research practices seem to be in violation of the criminal law, important light may be shed on the nature of the flaws with these practices. The criminal law generally reflects minimum standards of conduct all members of society are bound to respect; it is the ultimate means by which norms of social conduct are enforced.

As discussed above, Paul Kalb and Kristin Koehler have suggested that provisions of the U.S. federal *False Claims Act* have been and may be used to prosecute deception in research.[145] On the basis of the *False*

Claims Act, the Department of Justice has investigated cases where informed consent was inadequate and conflicts of interest were not disclosed.[146]

Following this approach, we believe it would be worth investigating ways in which provisions of the Canadian Criminal Code could apply in extreme cases of research misconduct. In the context of finder's fees, physicians who fail to disclose such fees to their patients could be charged with fraud under section 380(1) of the Code, a provision that Canadian courts have interpreted broadly.[147]

Section 380(1) of the Code provides for punishment on summary conviction, and prison terms ranging up to two years (where value of the subject of the offence is less than $5,000) and to ten years (where same value is greater than $5,000) for 'Every one who, by deceit, false-hood or other fraudulent means, whether or not it is a false pretence within the meaning of this Act, defrauds the public or any person, whether ascertained or not, of any property, money or valuable security or any service.'

In our view, a charge under section 380(1) might be brought in circumstances where a patient in need of treatment is referred by a physician to research, where that physician's financial interests are not disclosed to the patient, and where the patient's treatment suffers as a result. The Supreme Court of Canada, in *R. v. Gaetz*, held that it is necessary for fraud to be found that the victim be deprived of something to which she was or might have been entitled.[148] The patient in the circumstance we describe above is defrauded of standard treatment. Furthermore, the patient may not have assumed the risks and costs associated with research participation, had she known of the finder's fees, and thus had reason to question the grounds upon which her physician made the referral.

Physicians' failure to disclose their financial interests in research referrals is likely not often the result of deliberate, intentional dishonesty; nonetheless, they may be held accountable for fraud. In *R. v. Zlatic*, the Supreme Court of Canada held that any means used that could be characterized as dishonest by the objective standard of the reasonable person would suffice.[149] Furthermore, the physician need not make statements that mislead the patient into thinking that the referral is in her best interests. The Quebec Court of Appeal, in *R. v. Emond*, held that the fraudulent act may be an omission; in the circumstances we contemplate, the omission would be failure to disclose the fee.[150] The Supreme Court of Canada, in *R. v. Campbell*, held that the Crown, in making out a charge of fraud, must prove risk of prejudice to the victim's economic interests.[151] We suggest that it may not be difficult to make this out in many instances in which finder's fees are implicated. The victim may suffer costs associated with participation in research (e.g., time lost from work, travel and relocation expenses, etc.); she may also suffer significant costs if her medical condition worsens as a result of her participation in the research.

The courts have in the past held that there was fraud where the accused deceived the victim as to the existence of a conflict of interest, and thereby placed the victim's interests at risk. In *R. v. Knowles*, for example, the Ontario Court of Appeal found that '[t]he deceit practiced by the respondent placed him in a position where his personal interest might conflict with the interest of his employer ... and imperil the complainant's economic interests. The complainant was thus placed in a position of risk in which it would not have been placed if it had not been deceived as to the true state of affairs.'[152]

There also seem to be interesting parallels between the circumstances of another case, *R. v. Roy*, and those in which we suggest finder's fees may attract charges.[153] In *Roy*, the accused, a sales manager, was charged with fraud in connection with fees he collected for shipping cars. The fees ranged from two hundred to four thousand dollars above the actual cost of the shipping, and neither the accused's employer nor his customers were informed of the charge. The court found that Roy had defrauded his employer and his customers.

Similar reasoning could be employed in analysis of finder's fees. Finder's fees are often collected without the knowledge of either the employer or the patient. Both may suffer as a result. Academic and clinical centres may suffer economic loss as a result of loss of their employee's services; the patient may suffer loss of standard treatment and costs associated with research participation. Most interesting is that in *Roy*, the court found that the accused was an agent of his customers in making shipping arrangements for the cars. If the court found that such a special relationship existed in a commercial context, it is difficult to imagine that the fiduciary nature of the patient-physician relationship would not weigh heavily as they assess the behaviour of physicians who accept finder's fees for referral of their unsuspecting patients.

Discussion

We have reviewed the ethical issues and existing policy and law relating to the acceptance of finder's fees for referral of patients to research.

While detailed policy guidance is available both for review boards and physicians, it is inadequate to the task of protecting subjects from conflicts presented by finder's fees well hidden in the budgets of research studies and from the influence of other incentives associated with subject recruitment. We have suggested that in order fully to appreciate the seriousness and scope of the issues presented by finder's fees, the phenomenon must be situated within the wider context of the commercialization of research. The impact of finder's fees will only become more pronounced as commercial interests in research – and in particular in clinical trials – continue to grow. Future investigation and attempts to regulate finder's fees must take stock of the broad range of incentives influencing the recruitment of patients and the way in which these reflect more fundamental shifts in the research environment.

As has been discussed elsewhere, a variety of stakeholders must be involved in any effort to improve policy measures aimed at counteracting the negative impact of the commercialization of research, from regulatory agencies, funding agencies, academic institutions, and professional organizations to editors of medical journals and representatives of the pharmaceuticals industry.[154] Improved regulation and policy ought to provide prominent and detailed guidance on finder's fees.

Many academic institutions have worked in recent decades on developing conflict of interest policies and policies for the review of industry-sponsored clinical research contracts.[155] Some academic institutions also have policies expressly prohibiting finder's fees,[156] although it is often unclear what enforcement mechanisms and penalties exist and whether they may reasonably be expected to be effective. Furthermore, a 2000 U.S. national survey of policies on disclosure of conflicts of interest in research revealed that only three institutions had policies requiring the disclosure of conflicts of interest to research subjects and the IRB.[157] The study found additionally that for violations of these policies 'nonspecific penalties were common, and the application of penalties was uniformly discretionary.'[158] This survey and others like it indicate that most existing institutional conflict of interest policies contain significant flaws.[159] The variety of standards for the identification of conflicts, procedures for their resolution, and sanctions for policy violations undermines the transparency of the system and makes it hard to justify continued confidence that institutions are independently capable of dealing with this issue.

Institutional research ethics review should include rigorous scrutiny of the allocation of funds in study budgets. Contract specialists, budget analysts, and specialized conflict-of-interest committees, which in many institutions already do preliminary verification of the appropriateness of fees and other financial interests, should be asked to provide detailed budget analyses to IRB/REBs and host institutions. Research institutions and teaching hospitals should bind trial sponsors through contract to full and detailed disclosure of the financial arrangements among all trial sponsors, researchers, and those involved in subject recruitment. These institutions should also contract for the authority to intervene when these interests threaten to unduly influence scientific and ethical standards. Review boards should have access to information provided under contract by research sponsors, and they should have the authority to request further disclosure as necessary.

A crucial precondition for adequate oversight of conflicts of interest in research is that bodies responsible for oversight be structured and regulated in such a way as to be fully independent of the commercial interests whose encroachment they are to guard against. Meeting this precondition will, in our view, ultimately require a legislated regulatory structure for the review boards system, coupled with meaningful national oversight and specific legal sanctions. Other countries have recognized this need and have moved towards review boards mandated by legislation with strict territorial jurisdiction.[160] In the United States, the Senate is hearing arguments in support of federal legislative intervention that would provide uniform standards, centralized oversight of IRBs, and heavy civil penalties for individuals and institutions found to have violated research regulations. Members of the House and Senate, spearheaded by Senator Edward Kennedy, are in the process of working on such legislation.[161] Provisions of their draft Bill, entitled the *Research Revitalization Act of 2002*, look very promising.

The proposed *Research Revitalization Act* is based on the growing recognition in the United States that 'legislation is required to enhance the current system for protecting research participants.'[162] Among other things, the Act is expected to provide 'comprehensive protection' for subjects, 'effective oversight' of research and research review, and 'to prevent improper conflicts of interest by those conducting or providing for the ethical oversight of research.'[163] To the latter end, a number of provisions relating to conflicts of interest have been proposed. To begin with, standards for accreditation of IRBs are proposed, including a requirement that they demonstrate an ability to 'adequately insulate decisions of the Board from improper conflicts of interest' in order to be accredited, and to retain their accreditation.[164] If adopted and enforced, this provision would help to ensure that IRBs have the independence necessary to undertake meaningful scrutiny of conflicts of interest in research. The Act goes further to provide improved regulatory direction and enhanced authority to IRBs. These enhancements include a provision for the eventual promulgation of regulations governing 'payments for the recruitment or participation of human participants in covered research.'[165] It is to be hoped that these regulations will govern all aspects of subject recruitment, including payments to investigators, physicians, and other health professionals for their part in recruiting subjects. The most promising enhancements of the proposed Act relating to the regulation of conflicts of interest are contained in Title IV – Financial Conflicts of Interest. For our purposes, among the most important provisions in Title IV are those that require investigators and IRB members to disclose on an ongoing basis potential conflicts of interest to IRBs or institutional Conflict of Interest Committees;[166] require IRBs, absent specified 'compelling circumstances,' to withhold approval of protocols posing more than minimal risk to participants if an 'investigator directly participating' in the research has a significant investment, or receives significant income, from a financially interested research sponsor;[167] and, where the IRB finds compelling circumstances, require it to ensure that subjects will be adequately informed of the source of the conflict.[168] Importantly, the draft *Research Revitalization Act* also provides for adequate remedies in the event of violation of its requirements: an injunction will be the normal remedy, but for 'substantial' infractions, civil damages up to $250,000 may be awarded.[169]

It should be noted that some state legislators have forged ahead of the Senate in strengthening existing protections for research subjects. Maryland, for instance, has enacted a law that in effect compels all researchers in the state to comply with existing federal regulations, which otherwise apply only to some government-funded human subjects research.[170] It also allows for injunctive relief where these regulations are violated and forces IRBs to make their decisions available for scrutiny upon request.

Health Canada should consider these initiatives in its ongoing discussion of alternative governance structures for research involving human subjects. It is essential that we also work to ensure uniform protection of subjects under an independent review structure. This will require the development of legislation through which existing protections for human subjects are consolidated; standards for the accreditation and oversight of REBs are established; greater direction and authority is provided to REBs; and remedies are provided sufficient to deter researchers, host institutions, and sponsors from developing relationships that corrode the fiduciary physician-patient relationship.

While governments and professional organizations bear responsibility for improving relevant regulation and policy, in the end physicians and others involved in research must always be alert to the inherent tension between the ends of research and practice. They must be sensitive to the ways in which this tension may be exacerbated by commercial and personal financial interests and careful not to compromise their moral and legal obligations on account of these interests. The vigilance and integrity of individual health professionals is ultimately essential to ensuring that patient care is not compromised by personal and commercial financial interests in research. Through such vigilance, forces that threaten to undermine the integrity of the profession and public trust in the conduct of research may be counteracted. In the end, as in any other realm of social activity, in research those who fail to meet their legal obligations to others ought to be brought to account for their failures before the law. Better enforcement of existing professional and legal mechanisms, including the use of the criminal law where needed, will drive home the message that the integrity of the research process and the protection of human subjects are crucial societal values that are in need of better protection.

It would be wrong, however, to rely solely upon professional regulations and potential liability of individual investigators. As we indicated, there are significant structural pressures that push towards the use of financial recruitment incentives. If underlying structural problems are not addressed, some people will still be tempted by the lure of profit, notwithstanding the threat of significant sanctions. It is therefore important to refer to some radical and, in a way, simpler solutions that have been proposed to deal with the growing demise of scientific integrity and the growing impact of commercial interests on the conduct and outcome of medical research.[171]

Several commentators have argued that a fundamental change in the regulatory review of clinical trials is needed to separate those who design, conduct, and review research from those who have financial interests in the outcome. Sheldon Krimsky recommends the establishment of a new National Institute for Drug Testing (NIDT).[172] A company wishing to apply for approval of a new drug would negotiate an appropriate protocol with the NIDT, which would organize the clinical trial, using qualified drug assessment centres. Marcia Angell recommends that a similar institute be established within the National Institutes of Health.[173] In Canada, a report by Royal Commissioner Roy Romanow also supports the establishment of an independent National Drug Agency.[174]

If drug trials were more tightly monitored and conducted more independently of those with a direct interest in the fast approval of new drugs or devices, financial recruitment incentives could be controlled more effectively. In addition, a national drug testing agency would determine more strictly which clinical trials are appropriate and which are not. This might diminish the number of clinical trials being undertaken, thus decreasing the pressure to find enough research subjects.

These recommendations deserve attention, especially in light of the recent controversies surrounding the efficacy and safety of a variety of drugs such as SSRIs and pain-killers such as VIOXX. The establishment of a national drug-testing agency to coordinate and supervise the research that supports applications for approval of a new drug or medical device would not only lead to a better control of research practices such as the payment of recruitment incentives, it would also strengthen the integrity of the medical research scene itself.[175]

NOTES

This paper, slightly revised and updated, is reprinted with permission from the *Journal of Law, Medicine & Ethics*, where it first appeared in (2003) 31:3 at 398–418 as 'The Human Subjects Trade: Ethical and Legal Issues Surrounding Recruitment Incentives.' The authors thank Kevin Davis for his comments on an earlier draft of the paper; Sujit Choudhry for suggestions relating to professional regulations in Ontario; and Dominique Sprumont and colleagues at the Institut de Droit de la Santé of Neuchâtel for providing information on Swiss case law developments. They also thank two anonymous reviewers for the *Journal of Law, Medicine & Ethics* for their helpful comments. Research for this publication was supported by grants from the Ontario Genomics Institute (Genome Canada) and the Stem Cell Network (National Centres for Excellence).

1 Robert Whitaker, 'Lure of Riches Fuels Testing,' *Boston Globe,* 17 November 1998, A1; Kurt Eichenwald and Gina Kolata, 'Drug Trials Hide Conflicts for Doctors,' *New York Times,* 16 May 1999, §1, 1. See also Lori B. Andrews, 'Money Is Putting People at Risk in Biomedical Research,' *Chronicle of Higher Education* 46:27 (10 March 2000) B4.

2 Eichenwald and Kolata, 'Drug Trials Hide Conflicts for Doctors.'

3 Ibid.

4 Alice Dembner, 'Who's Protecting the Children? Drug Research Raises Concerns About Policy and Penalties' *Boston Globe,* 25 March 2001, A1.

5 U.S., Department of Health and Human Services, Office of Inspector General, *Recruiting Human Subjects: Pressures in Industry-Sponsored Clinical Research* (Boston: Office of Evaluation and Inspections, 2000) at 8, 25.

6 Few articles focus exclusively on recruitment incentives. See Stuart Lind, 'Finder's Fees for Research Subjects' (1990) 303 New Eng. J. Med. 192; Stuart Lind, 'Is the Practice of Offering Finder's Fees for Subject Recruitment Appropriate? Is the Practice Widespread or Unique to My Institution? What Is the Proper Role of the IRB? What Is the Role of the Institution?' (1990) 12:4 IRB: A Review of Human Subjects Research 6; Evan G. DeRenzo, 'Coercion in the Recruitment and Retention of Human Research Subjects, Pharmaceutical Industry Payments to Physician-Investigators, and the Moral Courage of the IRB' (2000) 22:2 IRB: A Review of Human Subjects Research 1; Paul B. Miller and Trudo Lemmens, 'Finder's Fees and Therapeutic Obligations' (2002) 5:1 Geriatrics and Aging 66; Timothy Caulfield and Glenn Griener, 'Conflicts of Interest in Clinical Research: Addressing the Issue of Physician Remuneration' (2002) 30 J.L. Med. & Ethics 305. Other articles do refer to some of the issues in varying degrees of detail. See, e.g., Rebecca Dresser, 'Payment to Research Participants: The Importance of Context' (2001) 1:2 American Journal of Bioethics 47; Mark A. Rothstein, 'Currents in Contemporary Ethics: The Role of IRBs in Research Involving Commercial Biobanks' (2002) 30 J.L. Med. & Ethics 105 at 106 and other articles cited below.

7 Jesse A. Goldner, 'Dealing with Conflicts of Interest in Biomedical Research: IRB Oversight as the Next Best Solution to the Abolition Approach' (2000) 28 J.L. Med. & Ethics 379 at 382.

8 See U.S. Department of Health and Human Services, *Recruiting Human Subjects: Pressures in Industry-Sponsored Clinical Research* at 16; U.S., Department of Health and Human Services, Office of Inspector General, *Recruiting Human Subjects: Sample Guidelines for Practice* (2000) 1 at 8. See also E. Fuller Torrey, 'The Going Rate on Shrinks: Big Pharma and the Buying of Psychia-

try' (2002) 13:13 The American Prospect. A study by Elizabeth A. Boyd and Lisa A. Bero, in which they analysed disclosures of financial ties with industry by researchers at the University of California, revealed that 34 per cent of disclosed relationships involved paid speaking engagements, providing speakers with annual revenues ranging between $200 and $20,000. See Elizabeth A. Boyd and Lisa A. Bero, 'Assessing Faculty Relationships with Industry: A Case Study' (2000) 184 J. Am. Med. Assoc. 2209 at 2211.

9 See Boyd and Bero, 'Assessing Faculty Relationships with Industry' at 2211–12 for a case analysis of such relationships. Boyd and Bero report that 33 per cent of disclosed relationships involved paid consulting, for which annual revenues ranged between $1,000 and $120,000.

10 U.S. Department of Health and Human Services, *Recruiting Human Subjects*: *Pressures in Industry-Sponsored Clinical Research* at 1, 15.

11 Robert P. Kelch, 'Maintaining the Public Trust in Clinical Research' (2002) 346 New Eng. J. Med. 285; Joseph B. Martin and Dennis L. Kasper, 'In Whose Best Interest? Breaching the Academic-Industrial Wall' (2000) 343 New Eng. J. Med. 1646; Marcia Angell, 'Is Academic Medicine for Sale?' (2000) 342 New Eng. J. Med. 1516; Steven Lewis et al., 'Dancing with the Porcupine: Rules for Governing the University-Industry Relationship' (2001) 165 Can. Med. Assoc. J. 783; Richard A. Rettig, 'The Industrialization of Clinical Research' (2000) 19 Health Affairs 129; and Karine Morin et al., 'Managing Conflicts of Interest in the Conduct of Clinical Trials' (2002) 287 J. Am. Med. Assoc. 78 at 78.

12 Morin et al., 'Managing Conflicts of Interest' at 78.

13 Marilynn Larkin, 'Clinical Trials: What Price Progress?' (1999) 354 Lancet 1534.

14 Morin et al., 'Managing Conflicts of Interest' at 78.

15 Morin et al., 'Managing Conflicts of Interest'; 'The Industrialization of Clinical Research.'

16 Larkin, 'Clinical Trials' at 1534.

17 Morin et al., 'Managing Conflicts of Interest' at 78; see also Thomas Bodenheimer, 'Uneasy Alliance: Clinician Investigators and the Pharmaceutical Industry' (2000) 342 New Eng. J. Med. 1539 at 1539.

18 Adil E. Shamoo, 'Adverse Events Reporting: The Tip of an Iceberg' (2001) 8 Accountability in Research 197.

19 It is hard to say how realistic this number is. Clearly, the United States leads Canada in research funding by a considerable margin. Furthermore, in the United States many may participate in research to obtain access to treatment.

20 *Regulations Amending the Food and Drug Regulations (1024 – Clinical Trials),* P.C. 2001-1042, C. Gaz. 2001.II.1116 at 1139.
21 Lewis et al., 'Dancing with the Porcupine' at 783.
22 Ibid.
23 Ibid.
24 Shamoo, 'Adverse Events Reporting' at 197.
25 Goldner, 'Dealing with Conflicts of Interest in Biomedical Research' at 382.
26 Bodenheimer, 'Uneasy Alliance' at 1539.
27 Ibid.
28 Donald W. Light and Joel Lexchin, 'Will Lower Drug Prices Jeopardize Drug Research?: A Policy Fact Sheet' (2004) 4:1 Am. J. Bioethics W1.
29 The issue of payment of subjects is clearly related to that of payment of finder's fees. Finder's fees are intended to attract researchers to recruitment activity; payments to subjects are intended to convince subjects to participate. We focus in this article on the pressure exercised on researchers and on how this affects their legal and ethical duties. For a discussion of payment of subjects, see Christine Grady, 'Money for Research Participation: Does It Jeopardize Informed Consent?' (2001) 1:2 Am. J. Bioethics 40 and commentaries; Trudo Lemmens and Carl Elliott, 'Guinea Pigs on the Payroll: The Ethics of Paying Research Subjects' (1999) 7 Accountability in Research 3.
30 Dembner, 'Who's Protecting the Children?'
31 Whitaker, 'Lure of Riches Fuels Testing.'
32 U.S. Department of Health and Human Services, *Recruiting Human Subjects: Pressures in Industry-Sponsored Clinical Research* at 13.
33 Bodenheimer, 'Uneasy Alliance' at 1539.
34 U.S. Department of Health and Human Services, *Recruiting Human Subjects: Pressures in Industry-Sponsored Clinical Research* at 18.
35 Goldner, 'Dealing with Conflicts of Interest' at 382. See also Bodenheimer, 'Uneasy Alliance' at 1541.
36 U.S., National Institutes of Health, *Conference on Human Subject Protection and Financial Conflicts of Interest* (conference transcript) (2000) at 45.
37 Bodenheimer, 'Uneasy Alliance' at 1540.
38 Rettig, 'The Industrialization of Clinical Research' at 138.
39 Ibid. at 139; U.S. Department of Health and Human Services, *Recruiting Human Subjects: Pressures in Industry-Sponsored Clinical Research* at 11.
40 Whitaker, 'Lure of Riches Fuels Testing.'
41 Ruth Macklin, cited in Larkin, 'Clinical Trials.'
42 See generally U.S. Department of Health and Human Services, *Recruiting Human Subjects: Pressures in Industry-Sponsored Clinical Research* at 20–6. See

also Donna Shalala, 'Protecting Research Subjects – What Must Be Done' (2000) 343 New Eng. J. Med. 808 at 808; and Morin et al., 'Managing Conflicts of Interest' at 80.

43 See note 1 above.

44 Supra note 36 at 14. See also Goldner, 'Dealing with Conflicts of Interest' at 381.

45 U.S. Department of Health and Human Services, *Recruiting Human Subjects: Pressures in Industry-Sponsored Clinical Research* at 25.

46 Personal communication from Dr Barry Goldlist to the author (TL) (10 December 2001).

47 Larkin, 'Clinical Trials' at 1534. See also Franklin G. Miller and Andrew F. Shorr, 'Ethical Assessment of Industry-Sponsored Clinical Trials: A Case Analysis' (2002) 121 CHEST 1337 at 1337.

48 See Julio S.G. Montaner, Michael V. O'Shaughnessy, and Martin T. Schechter, 'Industry-Sponsored Clinical Research: A Double-Edged Sword' (2001) 358 Lancet 1893; C. David Naylor, 'Early Toronto Experience with New Standards for Industry-Sponsored Clinical Research: A Progress Report' (2002) 166 Can. Med. Assoc. J. 453.

49 Bodenheimer, 'Uneasy Alliance' at 1541–2. See also Frank Davidoff, 'Between the Lines: Navigating the Uncharted Territory of Industry-Sponsored Research' (2002) 21 Health Affairs 235, and 'Look, No Strings: Publishing Industry-Funded Research' Editorial (2001) 165 Can. Med. Assoc. J. 733.

50 Bodenheimer, 'Uneasy Alliance' at 1541–2.

51 U.S. Department of Health and Human Services, *Recruiting Human Subjects: Pressures in Industry-Sponsored Clinical Research* at 17.

52 See, e.g., reports on the Nancy Olivieri affair: Report to the Board of Trustees of the Hospital for Sick Children, *Clinical Trials of L1 (Deferiprone) at the Hospital for Sick Children: A Review of Facts and Circumstances* (8 December 1998), http://www.sickkids.ca/l1trials/revcontents.asp; Jon Thompson, Patricia Baird, and Jocelyn Downie, *The Olivieri Report: The Complete Text of the Report of the Independent Inquiry Commissioned by the Canadian Association of University Teachers* (Toronto: James Lorimer, 2001); Arnold Naimark, Bartha M. Knoppers, and Frederick H. Lowy, 'Commentary on Selected Aspects of the Report of the Committee of Inquiry on the Case of Dr Olivieri, the Hospital for Sick Children, the University of Toronto, and Apotex Inc.' (December 2001), http://www.sickkids.on.ca/MediaRoom/CAUTfinal2ed.pdf; Jon Thompson, Patricia Baird, and Jocelyn Downie, 'Supplement to the Report of the Committee of Inquiry on the Case Involving Dr Nancy Olivieri, the Hospital for Sick Children, the University of

Toronto, and Apotex Inc' (30 January 2002), http://www.doctorsinteg-rity.org/media/CAUT_supplement.doc.

53 Goldner, 'Dealing with Conflicts of Interest' at 385.

54 For an interesting argument on how payment of subjects affects the moral status and social conception of research participation, see Tod Chambers, 'Participation as Commodity, Participation as Gift' (2001) 1:2 Am. J. Bioeth-ics 48.

55 R. Orlowski and L. Wateska, 'The Effects of Pharmaceutical Firm Entice-ments on Physician Prescribing Patterns' (1992) 102 CHEST 270.

56 See generally Goldner, 'Dealing with Conflicts of Interest' at 390; and Kath-leen Cranley Glass and Trudo Lemmens, 'Conflict of Interest and Commer-cialization of Biomedical Research: What Is the Role of Research Ethics Review?' in Timothy Caulfield and Bryn Williams-Jones, eds., *The Commer-cialization of Genetic Research: Ethical, Legal and Policy Issues* (New York: Klu-wer, 1999), 79 at 79.

57 Goldner, 'Dealing with Conflicts of Interest' at 390; Janet Fleetwood, 'Con-flicts of Interest in Clinical Research: Advocating for Patient-Subjects' (2001) 8 Widener L. Symp. J. 105 at 112.

58 U.S., Food and Drug Administration, *Information Sheets: Guidance for Institu-tional Review Boards and Clinical Investigators* (1998).

59 U.S. Department of Health and Human Services, *Recruiting Human Subjects: Pressures in Industry-Sponsored Clinical Research* at 26.

60 Ibid.

61 The DHHS regulations are at 42 C.F.R. Subpart F; the FDA regulations at 21 C.F.R. Parts 54, 312, 314, 320, 330, 601, 807, 812, 814, and 860.

62 See Association of American Medical Colleges, Task Force on Financial Conflicts of Interest in Clinical Research, *Protecting Subjects, Preserving Trust, Promoting Progress: Policy and Guidelines for the Oversight of Individual Financial Conflict of Interest in Human Subjects Research* (2001), http:// www.aamc.org/members/coitf/start.htm at 5–6. The shortcomings of the regulations are also recognized in U.S., Department of Health and Human Services, *Final Guidance Document*, http://www.hhs.gov/ohrp/ humansubjects/finreltn/fguid.pdf [*Final Guidance Document*].

63 See Shalala, 'Protecting Research Subjects' at 810.

64 *Final Guidance Document*; U.S., Department of Health and Human Services, Draft, *Financial Relationships and Interests in Research Involving Human Sub-jects: Guidance for Human Subject Protection* 68 Fed. Reg. 15,456 (2003).

65 See Rick Weiss, 'New HHS Panel Makeup Draws Ire of Patient Advocates,' *Washington Post*, 5 January 2003, A09.

66 Task Force on Financial Conflicts of Interest in Clinical Research, *Protecting*

Subjects; Association of American Medical Colleges, Task Force on Financial Conflict of Interest in Clinical Research, Institutional Conflict of Interest, *Protecting Subjects, Preserving Trust, Promoting Progress II: Principles and Recommendations for Oversight of an Institution's Financial Interests in Human Subjects Research* (Association of American Medical Colleges, 2001).
67 *Regulations Amending the Food and Drug Regulations (1024 – Clinical Trials)* at 1131.
68 Bernard M. Dickens, 'Conflict of Interest in Canadian Health Care Law' (1995) 21 Am. J.L. and Med. 259 at 274.
69 Medical Research Council of Canada, Natural Sciences and Engineering Research Council of Canada, and Social Sciences and Humanities Research Council of Canada, *Tri-Council Policy Statement* (Ottawa: Minister of Supply and Services, 1998) at Art. 4.1. In the section dealing with clinical trials, the *Policy Statement* also explicitly requires REBs to examine the budgets of clinical trials (see Art. 7.3).
70 Ibid. at Art. 7.3.
71 Ibid. at Art. 2.6(e).
72 For more on the limits on the responsibility of REBs, see Dale Keiger and Sue De Pasquale, 'Trials and Tribulation' *Johns Hopkins Magazine* 54:1 (February 2002), http://www.jhu.edu/~jhumag/0202web/trials.html.
73 For similar arguments in consideration of the U.S. system, see Fleetwood, 'Conflicts of Interest in Clinical Research.'
74 See generally George Grob, 'Institutional Review Boards: A Time for Reform' (Testimony before the Committee on Government Reform and Oversight, 11 June 1998) (Washington, DC: Office of Inspector General, Department of Health and Human Services, 1998) [*Time for Reform*]; Greg Koski, 'Risks, Benefits, and Conflicts of Interest in Human Research: Ethical Evolution in the Changing World of Science' (2000) 28 J.L. Med. and Ethics 330; Shalala, 'Protecting Research Subjects' at 809.
75 Trudo Lemmens and Benjamin Freedman, 'Ethics Review for Sale? Conflict of Interest and Commercial Research Review Boards' (2000) 78 Milbank Quarterly 547.
76 *Regulations Amending the Food and Drug Regulations* at 1143, 1132.
77 See Lorraine E. Ferris, 'Industry-Sponsored Pharmaceutical Trials and Research Ethics Boards: Are They Cloaked in Too Much Secrecy?' (2002) 166 Can. Med. Assoc. J. 1279 at 1279.
78 Charles Weijer, 'Placebo Trials and Tribulations' (2002) 166 Can. Med. Assoc. J. 603.
79 *Tri-Council Policy Statement* at Art. 7.4 (discussing placebo controls).
80 *Time for Reform*; U.S., Department of Health and Human Services, Office of

Inspector General, *Institutional Review Boards: The Emergence of Independent Boards* (Boston: Office of Evaluation and Inspections, 1998); U.S., Department of Health and Human Services, Office of Inspector General, *Institutional Review Boards: Their Role in Reviewing Approved Research* (Boston: Office of Evaluation and Inspections, 1998); U.S., Department of Health and Human Services, Office of Inspector General, *Institutional Review Boards: Promising Approaches* (Boston: Office of Evaluation and Inspections, 1998); U.S., National Bioethics Advisory Commission, *Ethical and Policy Issues in Research Involving Human Participants* (Bethesda, MD: National Bioethics Advisory Commission, 2001); Mildred K. Cho and Paul Billings, 'Conflict of Interest and Institutional Review Boards' (1997) 45 J. Investigative Med. 154.

81 Trudo Lemmens and Alison Thompson, 'Non-Institutional Research Review Boards in North America: A Critical Appraisal and Comparison with IRBs' (2001) 23:2 IRB: A Review of Human Subjects Research 1.

82 Lemmens and Freedom, 'Ethics Review for Sale?'; Cho and Billings, '*Conflict of Interest*'; Leslie Francis, 'IRBs and Conflicts of Interest,' in Roy G. Spece, David S. Shimm and Allen E. Buchanan, eds., *Conflicts of Interest in Clinical Practice and Research* (New York: Oxford University Press, 1996), 418.

83 Ferris, 'Industry-Sponsored Pharmaceutical Trials' at 1279.

84 Marie Hirtle, Trudo Lemmens, and Dominique Sprumont, 'A Comparative Analysis of Research Ethics Review Mechanisms and the ICH Good Clinical Practice Guideline' (2000) 7 Eur. J. Health L. 265.

85 See Cho and Billings, 'Conflict of Interest' at 155; Glass and Lemmens, 'Conflict of Interest.'

86 Lemmens and Freedman, 'Ethics Review for Sale?'

87 See Cho and Billings, 'Conflict of Interest' at 156. See also Fleetwood, 'Conflicts of Interest in Clinical Research' at 111.

88 See generally, Hirtle, Lemmens, and Sprumont, 'A Comparative Analysis.'

89 Swiss Bundesgerichts, Second Public Law Division (4 July 2003), *Freiburger Ethik-Kommission International v. Regierungsrat des Kantons Basel-Landschaft* (2A.450/2002), http://wwwsrv.bger.ch/cgi-bin/AZA/MapProcessorCGI _AZA?mapfile=pull/ConvertDocFrameCGI.map&r i=fr&lang=fr&ds =AZA_pull&d=04.07.2003_2A.450%2f2002&pa=1%7e2a%2b4 50%2b2002 %4073%7e& [Translated by author TL]. A commentary on this case can be found in Alfred Jost, 'Freiburger Ethik-Kommission International c. Bâle-Campagne' *Revue suisse de droit de la santé* 1 (Sept. 2003) 13.

90 782 A.2d 807 (Md. 2001), recons. denied (2001).

91 Dickens, 'Conflict of Interest at 274.

92 *Tri-Council Policy Statement* at Art. 4.1.
93 Canadian Medical Association, *Physicians and the Pharmaceutical Industry* (Ottawa: Canadian Medical Association, 2001).
94 Ibid. ¶ 3.
95 Ibid. ¶ 11.
96 American Medical Association, Council on Ethical and Judicial Affairs, 'Conflicts of Interest: Biomedical Research' [opinion E-8.031] in *Code of Medical Ethics: Current Opinions* (Chicago: American Medical Association, 2000).
97 Ibid.
98 American Medical Association, Council on Ethical and Judicial Affairs, 'Fee Splitting: Referrals to Health Care Facilities [opinion E-6.03]' in *Code of Medical Ethics: Current Opinions* (Chicago: American Medical Association, 2000).
99 Ibid.
100 American Medical Association, Council on Ethical and Judicial Affairs, *Finder's Fees: Payment for the Referral of Patients to Clinical Research Studies* (Chicago: American Medical Association, 1994).
101 Ibid.
102 *False Claims Act*, 31 U.S.C. § 3729(a) (2001).
103 *Anti-Kickback Statute*, 42 U.S.C. § 1320a–1327b (201).
104 Paul E. Kalb and Kristin G. Koehler, 'Legal Issues in Scientific Research' (2002) 287 J. Am. Med. Assoc. 85.
105 Ibid. at 86.
106 Ibid. at 87–9.
107 45 C.F.R. § 46.
108 21 C.F.R. § 50.
109 42 C.F.R. § 50.604.
110 Kalb and Koehler, 'Legal Issues in Scientific Research' at 89.
111 Ibid. at 86, 89.
112 Ibid. at 89.
113 Sujit Choudhry, Adalsteinn D. Brown, and Niteesh K. Choudhry, 'Unregulated Private Markets for Health Care in Canada? Kickbacks to Physicians and Physician Self-Referral in Canada' (2004) 170 Can. Med. Assoc. J. 1115.
114 *Medicine Act, 1991*, S.O. 1991, c. 30, *Professional Misconduct Regulations*, O. Reg. 856/93, amended to R.R.O. 53/95. We are indebted to Sujit Choudhry for bringing these provisions to our attention.
115 *Health Professions Procedural Code*, being Schedule II to the *Regulated Health Professions Act, 1991*, R.S.O. 1991, c. 18.
116 *Medicine Act, 1991* at Part IV.

117 For a short overview of the law on this issue, see Ellen I. Picard and Gerald B. Robertson, *Legal Liability of Doctors and Hospitals in Canada*, 3rd ed. (Toronto: Carswell, 1996) at 149–52; Kathleen Cranley Glass and Trudo Lemmens, 'Research Involving Humans,' in Jocelyn Downie, Timothy Caulfield, and Colleen Flood, eds., *Canadian Health Law and Policy*, 2nd ed. (Markham, ON: Butterworths, 2002), 459 at 493–7.

118 *Reibl v. Hughes*, [1980] 2 S.C.R. 880.

119 Ibid.

120 *Hopp v. Lepp*, [1980] 2 S.C.R. 192.

121 Picard and Robertson, *Legal Liability*, at 484.

122 Ibid.

123 See Dickens, 'Conflict of Interest.'

124 *Halushka v. University of Saskatchewan* (1965), 53 D.L.R. (2d) 436 at 443–4.

125 Ibid. at 444.

126 [1989] R.J.Q. 731 (Sup. Ct.).

127 *Moore v. The Regents of the University of California*, 793 P.2d 479 (Cal. 1990).

128 Ibid. at 483.

129 Ibid.

130 See Dickens, 'Conflict of Interest' at 273.

131 Marc A. Rodwin, 'Strains in the Fiduciary Metaphor: Divided Physician Loyalties and Obligations in a Changing Health Care System' (1995) 21 Am. J.L. and Med. 241 at 243–4.

132 *Norberg v. Wynrib*, [1992] 92 D.L.R. (4th) 449. See also Dickens, 'Conflict of Interest' at 261–2.

133 *Norberg v. Wynrib* at 486.

134 Ibid. at 487.

135 Ibid. at 486.

136 Ibid. at 489.

137 Ernest J. Weinrib, 'Restitutionary Damages as Corrective Justice' (2000) 1:1 Theor. Inq. L. 1 at 33.

138 *Whiten v. Pilot Insurance Co.* (2002), 209 D.L.R. (4th) 257 at 274.

139 Dickens, 'Conflict of Interest' at 264.

140 Rodwin, 'Strains in the Fiduciary Metaphor' at 246.

141 Ibid.

142 Ibid.

143 Fleetwood, 'Conflicts of Interest' at 109.

144 Picard and Robertson, *Legal Liability* at 484.

145 Kahl and Koehler, 'Legal Issues in Scientific Research.'

146 Ibid. at 88.

147 See Kevin Davis and Julian Roy, 'Fraud in the Canadian Courts: An

Unwarranted Expansion of the Scope of the Criminal Sanction' (1998) 30 Can. Bus. L.J. 210.

148 *R. v. Gaetz*, [1993] 3 S.C.R. 645.

149 *R. v. Zlatic*, [1993] 2 S.C.R. 29. See also *R. c. Lajoie*, [1999] J.Q. no 416 (C.A.).

150 *R. c. Emond*, [1997] A.Q. no. 1581 (C.A.).

151 *R. v. Campbell*, [1986] 2 S.C.R. 376.

152 *R. v. Knowles* (1979), 51 C.C.C. (2d) 237 at 241 (Ont. C.A.).

153 *R. v. Roy* (1994), 70 O.A.C. 127; for an interesting discussion of the ramifications of this case, see Davis and Roy, 'Fraud in the Canadian Courts' at 219–22.

154 David Korn, 'Conflicts of Interest in Biomedical Research' (2000) 284 J. Am. Med. Assoc. 2234. See Morin et al., 'Managing Conflicts of Interests' at 81–3; Rettig, 'The Industrialization of Clinical Research' at 140–3; Lewis et al., 'Dancing with the Porcupine.'

155 Naylor, 'Early Toronto Experience'; Lewis et al., 'Dancing with the Porcupine'; Mildred K. Cho et al., 'Policies on Faculty Conflicts of Interest at US Universities' (2000) 284 J. Am. Med. Assoc. 2237.

156 See, e.g. University of Toronto Faculty of Medicine, *Offer and Acceptance of Finder's Fees for the Recruitment of Research Subjects*, http://www.facmed .utoronto.ca/English/Policy-On-The-Offer-And-Acceptance-Of-Finders-Fees-Or-Completion-Fees-In-Research-Involving-Human-Subjects.html; University of Washington, *Policy Prohibiting the Use of Enrolment Incentives in Human Subjects Research*, http://www.washington.edu/research/osp/ forms/enrolmentincentives .pdf; University of Rochester Office of Research and Project Administration, *University of Rochester Policy on Enrolment Incentive Payments by or to University Clinical Trial Researchers*, http:// www.rochester.edu/ORPA/policies/incenpay.pdf; University of Tennessee, *Finder's Fees*, http://www.utmem.edu/policies/w932_document _show.php?p=237; Wayne State University, *Finder's Fees*, http:// www.hic.wayne.edu/hicpol/finders.htm. See also S. Van McCrary et al., 'A National Survey of Policies on Disclosure of Conflicts of Interest in Biomedical Research' (2000) 323 New Eng. J. Med. 1621.

157 McCrary et al., 'National Survey of Policies.'

158 Ibid. at 1623.

159 Ibid.; Bernard Lo, Leslie E. Wolf, and Abiona Berkeley, 'Conflict-of-Interest Policies for Investigators in Clinical Trials' (2000) 343 New Eng. J. Med. 1616; Cho et al., 'Policies on Faculty Conflicts of Interest'; Boyd and Bero, 'Assessing Faculty Relationships with Industry.'

160 See Hirtle, Lemmens, and Sprumont, 'Comparative Analysis.'

161 J.W. Schomisch, 'Senate Panel Told Federal Agency Needed for Human

Protection in Clinical Trials' *RAPS News* (24 April 2002), http://www.raps.org/news/senate04232002.cfm. See also Shalala, 'Protecting Research Subjects' at 809.

162 U.S., *Research Revitalization Act of 2002* (Discussion draft), 107th Cong. (2002) at § 2(a)(14).

163 Ibid. at § 2(b)(1–3)

164 Ibid. at tit. II, §§ 201(e)(2)(c), (f)(2).

165 Ibid. at tit. III, §§ 301(a)(1–2).

166 Ibid. at tit. IV, §§ 401(a)(1–3).

167 Ibid. at tit. IV, §§ 401(b)(1), (c).

168 Ibid. at tit. IV, § 401(d).

169 Ibid. at tit. V, §§ 501(a), (e).

170 U.S., H.D. 917, 143d Sess., Md. 2002.

171 For a detailed discussion of how the various regulatory mechanisms in the context of research fail to protect scientific integrity, see Trudo Lemmens, 'Leopards in the Temple: Restoring Integrity to the Commercialized Research Scene' (2004) 32 J.L. Med. and Ethics 641.

172 See Sheldon Krimsky, *Science in the Private Interest: Has the Lure of Profit Corrupted Biomedical Research?* (Lanham, MD: Rowman and Littlefield, 2003) at 229.

173 Commission on the Future of Health Care in Canada, *Building on Values: The Future of Health Care in Canada, Final Report* (2002) esp. at 199–210, http://www.hc-sc.gc.ca/english/pdf/romanow/pdfs/HCC_Final _Report.pdf.

174 See Marcia Angell, *The Truth About the Pharmaceutical Industry: How They Deceive Us and What to Do About It* (New York: Random House, 2004) at 244–7.

175 For more detailed discussion of these proposed solutions, see Lemmens, 'Leopards in the Temple' at 652ff.

PART THREE

Liability

8 Bringing Research into Therapy: Liability Anyone?[1]

MARY M. THOMSON

Gene therapy, better described as gene transfer research, is a technique used to correct defective genes responsible for disease development. The scientific community has promoted the potential of gene therapy for the past thirty years, and clinical trials have been ongoing for more than a decade. Yet there have been troubling developments and heart-breaking stories as this science moves from the laboratory to the clinic, from research to therapy, and from the theoretical to the practical. Because the promise of gene transfer research is so great, the setbacks seem enormously discouraging. Where the gap between expectation and outcome is marked, those harmed by an outcome will look increasingly to litigation as means of seeking redress.

In the past, research activities have not been the target of liability claims. Lawsuits against researchers have been few. The number and creativity of such claims is increasing, however, and since many of the pharmaceutical companies and universities that fund such research are located in the United States, litigation is often brought there with commensurately high damage awards. Lawsuits can now be expected in other countries where research has been undertaken: litigation has always fuelled more litigation.

The impact of threatened and successful lawsuits has made the research community anxious about its work being attacked in the courts. Several recent and highly publicized cases have addressed injuries sustained during clinical trials which were conducted at major academic institutions. Sponsors, researchers/investigators, Research Ethics Boards (REBs), known in the States as Institutional Review Boards (IRBs), academic and hospitals boards, and even patient advocates, previously thought to be relatively immune from litigation, have been put on notice that they are increasingly at risk of being named in lawsuits arising out of gene transfer trials. This chapter will address the legal framework within which adverse outcomes will be judged, as gene transfer moves from research to treatment.

I. Background

The field of gene therapy has come a long way over the past thirty years. In most gene transfer studies, a 'normal' gene is inserted into the genome to replace the 'abnormal' disease-causing gene. A carrier molecule or vector is used to deliver the therapeutic gene to the patient's target cells. Such vectors include retroviruses, adenoviruses, adeno-associated viruses, and herpes simplex virus. There are also non-viral delivery systems, including the direct introduction of therapeutic DNA to the target cells, and researchers are experimenting with the introduction of a forty-seventh (artificial) chromosome to target cells.[1]

There is a massive scientific literature on the topic of gene transfer research, mostly pertaining to studies with non-human subjects. The development of gene transfer has coincided with a maturation of the entire biotechnology sector. Gene transfer is but one of the areas in which industry-academia partnerships have become the norm, and entire corporations have been set up to finance gene transfer projects. A great deal is riding on the promise of gene transfer research, quite apart from medical progress or therapeutic benefit. Undoubtedly, this research will continue to be pursued and hopefully, one day it will deliver on its promise. In the meantime, however, gene transfer trials have garnered unwanted attention due to certain adverse outcomes.

In January 2003, the U.S. Food and Drug Administration (FDA) placed a temporary halt on all gene transfer trials using retroviral vectors in the blood stream.[2] This action was taken after the second of two French children developed a leukemia-like condition following gene therapy for X-linked severe combined immunodeficiency disease (X-SCID), known as 'bubble-boy' disease. After a decade of research and seemingly unblemished success,[3] researchers were devastated when first one boy in August 2002 and then another boy the following December presented with a leukemia-like cancer, possibly related to the use of the retroviral vectors.

Earlier disillusionment had come in September 1999, with the unexpected death of a healthy eighteen-year-old research participant, Jesse Gelsinger, while participating in a gene transfer trial at the University of Pennsylvania (see chapter 1). This case was the subject of litigation brought shortly after Jesse's death. *Gelsinger v. Trustees of the University of Pennsylvania* was resolved in November 2000 by way of a multi-million-dollar settlement. The case highlights many of the legal issues raised by gene transfer, including, but not limited to, informed consent, conflict of interest, and the effectiveness of regulatory safeguards in general.

In Canada, James Dent was diagnosed with brain cancer and given only ten months to live. He enrolled in a gene transfer trial in April 1997. Like Jesse Gelsinger, Dent died unexpectedly early in the experiment, although his death did not come to public attention until the spring of 2000. Several problems with the conduct of the research have since come to light. This case too raises issues of informed consent,[4] conflict of interest, and the standard of care provision in the context of research.[5]

The setbacks of these three cases have deflated much of the enthusiasm for gene transfer research found a decade ago. Using the Gelsinger and Dent cases as examples, this chapter will analyse civil liability for gene transfer under traditional principles of the common law. What legal framework would be applied if any of these cases came before a Canadian court today?[6] Given the increasing likelihood that litigation will also be brought in Canada to address adverse outcomes from clinical trials and gene transfer, comments will also be offered on proactive strategies for sponsors, researchers/investigators, REB/IRBs, and academic and hospital boards to safeguard their interests and, ideally, to reduce the risk of their own civil liability.

II. The Legal Framework

Negligence

A claim for damages for wrongful death or injury in a gene therapy trial would be framed in breach of contract and under the common law tort of negligence. To meet the test for negligence, 'the plaintiff must prove that any injury sustained was caused by the breach of a duty of care owed by the defendant(s) to the plaintiff. A breach would be judged by a failure to meet the appropriate standard of care.'[8] The onus on the plaintiff, strictly speaking, is therefore threefold:

1. to establish that the defendant owed a duty of care to the plaintiff;

2. to establish that the defendant breached that duty by falling short of the standard of care expected; and
3. to establish that that failure to meet the standard of care expected caused the injury suffered.

The principles of negligence will be expanded upon below. Plaintiffs are likely to cite negligence in:

1. the design of the research study;
2. the conduct and management of the research study;
3. a failure to provide adequate informed consent by warning of risks and side effects; and
4. a failure to provide proper medical care to the patient during the therapy by
   a) failing to evaluate a pre-existing medical condition;
   b) failing to diagnose a developing medical condition; and
   c) failing to treat a presenting medical condition through the course of the gene therapy.[9]

When a claim is brought in negligence in the context of gene transfer, the plaintiffs will make the following three allegations. First, that the sponsor, the researcher/investigator, the research institution, and the REB or IRB each failed to meet the standard of care expected of them in the design and conduct of the research protocol. Second, that they failed to meet the standard of care in selecting the plaintiff as a suitable subject for the proposed gene transfer trial. And third, that they failed to monitor the plaintiff's underlying medical status or to treat his or her developing condition in the course of the trial.

The case against each of the defendants will be based primarily on expert testimony identifying how and to what extent the defendants, individually and collectively, failed to meet the standard of care expected of them.

Evidence with respect to the standard of care will also be drawn from the regulatory scheme. Since the late 1990s, the potential liability of individual researchers must be considered in the context of two important 'rule sets' for clinical trials. The first of these is found in amendments to the *Food and Drugs Act* and its Regulations. In June 2001, the Parliament of Canada enacted the *Regulations Amending the Food and Drug Regulations (1024 – Clinical Trials)* to govern the 'sale and importation of drugs for use in human clinical trials.'[10] These provisions address the design and conduct of the research.

The second rule set is the earlier development of a policy statement on research in Canada, the *Tri-Council Policy Statement (TCPS)*.[11] In 1998, the three primary councils responsible for funding research in Canada released the *TCPS* to aid in the protection of human participants in research.[12] If researchers do not comply with the *TCPS*, funding may be withdrawn.

Both of these rule sets rely heavily for their implementation on the process for review of research ethics currently in place in Canada. Although not determinative of negligence, these rule sets, when taken together, provide a good indication of the expected standard of care to be met in the context of gene therapy trials. Accordingly, they are instructive in any analysis of negligence.

Informed Consent

It is also to be expected that researchers will meet with allegations of conflict of interest and a breach of fiduciary duties as elements of any negligence claim arising out of gene therapy.[13] Indeed, the most significant element of any negligence claim in the field of gene research or therapy is likely to be that of inadequate informed consent. The law imposes a heavy burden on researchers to provide informed consent to subjects in clinical trials or early therapy.

THE STANDARD IN THE RESEARCH SETTING
The requirement for fully informed consent in a research or new therapies situation is high for at least three reasons.

First, the knowledge base about the perceived risks and benefits of the research or therapy lies almost exclusively with the researchers. In the early stages of gene therapy, the data will not be known widely or readily available to the patients. (Information now available about the Gelsinger and Dent cases indicates that the requirement for fully informed consent was not adequate in either case.)

Second, proof of failure to meet the requirement of informed consent presents the most clear-cut means of potentially establishing liability in negligence against the co-defendants.

Third, as suggested above, the high standard of informed consent raises the issue of conflict of interest with alarming clarity.

In *Reibl v. Hughes*,[14] the Supreme Court of Canada established the standard of care for disclosure necessary to satisfy informed consent in the context of medical care. In order for a patient to provide his or her lawfully secured consent, the patient must be fully informed of all material risks that a reasonable patient, similarly situated, would want to know. The test applied in medical care cases has matured into that of the 'modified reasonable objective' test.

The standard for disclosure is far higher, however, for persons consenting to research. Although it is a forty-year-old precedent, *Halushka v. University of Saskatchewan*[15] remains the leading case addressing the conduct of medical research in Canada. In that case, Justice Hall stated with respect to the requirement for informed consent:

> There can be no exceptions to the ordinary requirements of disclosure in the case of research as there may well be in ordinary medical practice ... The example of risks being properly hidden from a patient when it is important that he should not worry can have no application in the field of research. *The subject of medical experimentation is entitled to a full and frank disclosure of all the facts, probabilities and opinions, which a reasonable man might be expected to consider before giving his consent.'*[16]

This 'full and frank disclosure' language was reproduced in the *Tri-Council Policy Statement.*[17]

The sentiment in *Halushka* was echoed in a more recent decision from the Quebec Superior Court in *Weiss v. Solomon.*[18] In *Weiss*, the court referred to the duty to inform as 'the most exacting possible.' Relevant information should include 'the revelation of all risks,' even 'those which are rare or remote and especially those which may entail serious consequences.'[19] There is general consensus that these passages embody a higher standard for informed consent than that provided for medical care. Any argument to the contrary has so far fallen short.[20]

Informed consent is intended to reinforce the autonomy of the prospective research participant or his legal representative. For the protection of those involved in a clinical trial or in gene therapy, no patient or subject should participate in either clinical research or early gene therapy without being provided with full and frank informed consent. The question in litigation will centre on the degree of informed consent necessary to satisfy the test of 'the most exacting possible' information.

As a general proposition, the information provided through informed consent should contain:

1. a statement that the study involves research;
2. an explanation of the purposes of that research;
3. a description of the research procedures to be followed, including an identification of any procedures considered to be experimental (i.e., a description of the methods and means by which the study will be conducted);
4. a description of any foreseeable risks including a description, if available, of the relative weighting of such risks;
5. a description of alternatives to the proposed therapy;
6. a description of the duration of the subject's participation; and
7. responses to any questions asked by the proposed subject.[21]

In the process of providing informed consent, the researcher should be aware of the following safeguards to avoid any suggestion of coercion or undue influence to participate in the research or gene therapy:

1. the subject should provide a statement specifying that all participation is completely voluntary;
2. the subject should be given adequate time to consider whether or not to participate in the proposed research;
3. all information should be provided in a language and manner familiar to the subject; the subject must have sufficient comprehension of the elements of the research to enable him or her to make an informed choice about participating;
4. there should be an undertaking that the researcher will provide study participants with relevant information throughout the duration of the study, particularly information about adverse events, any medical conditions that arise in the subject or other participants in the study, and any change in the participants' pre-existing medical condition that arises while participating in the study; and
5. disclosure must be made of any conflict of interest the researcher may have with furtherance of the study.[22]

While it is true that informed consent is the process of providing material information to the subject or his or her legal representative,[23] it is important to ensure that an informed consent form is signed freely and without any undue influence or duress; in other words, in a fully autonomous way. The form should contain no exculpatory language by which the subject waives any legal rights.

THE 'FULLY AUTONOMOUS RATIONAL DECISION-MAKER'

Despite these comments, the 'fully autonomous rational decision-maker' remains something of a fiction,[24] particularly in the context of research. Prospective research participants often come to a research team looking for hope when there is no hope left, or looking to help others when they themselves understand that they will not be cured. James Dent and Jesse Gelsinger embodied those aspirations. This measure of vulnerability and altruism adds further credence to the higher standard for disclosure in the research setting.

The Gelsinger and Dent cases provide a useful framework within which to consider the adequacy of the informed consent given, especially since in both cases, the research protocol had received approval from the relevant institutional ethical review body.

In the Gelsinger case, the seventeen human participants who preceded Jesse Gelsinger did not suffer adverse consequences from the gene therapy. The plaintiffs alleged, however, that monkeys had endured harmful effects from the same adenovirus vector as that which was used on Jesse and alleged that this was not mentioned before consent was given. In appropriate circumstances, evidence from animal models should be disclosed as part of the informed consent process in research trials.[25] In the earlier stages of a clinical trial, there will be less experience with human subjects. The less the experience with human subjects, the higher the obligation will be to disclose information about animal trials. Even using the modified reasonable person test, one could easily anticipate circumstances in which the human subject would want to know what had occurred in the animal trials.

In the Dent case, as the facts have been reported, James Dent had signed a consent form to participate in the research study. The consent form given to Mr Dent was not the form that the U.S. regulators had approved, which disclosed certain adverse event information. The version given to Mr Dent only warned that he would probably experience some flu-like symptoms.[26] The consent form he signed did not disclose that there was a risk of death associated with the intervention. Moreover, there was no disclosure that other individuals, who had previously taken part in a similar trial, had suffered 'serious adverse events.' In fact, seventeen of thirty participants had been so affected.

Of note, Mr Dent was not told that there had been a death in the United States during the course of his participation in the study. This omission was despite the fact that Mr Dent had made specific marginal notes on the consent form he signed, next to the assurance given to him by the researchers and the sponsor drug company that any new information about this therapy would be communicated to him.[27] An obligation to provide ongoing information during a research or investigational study is consistent with the case law[28] and the *Tri-Council Policy Statement*.[29] A researcher's failure to disclose material adverse events from past trials, whether on animals or humans, or to disclose material adverse events learned in the course of the clinical trial itself, will more likely than not be found to be a breach of the standard of care with respect to adequate disclosure.

A research participant always has the right to withdraw from a research project at any stage and without any penalty regarding treatment. Informing participants of this right is, in theory, part of the informed consent process.[30] Insofar as it could be established that James Dent was not given the information he was entitled to have, and in light of the fact that he had specifically requested receiving such information, his personal representatives would have a strong argument that he was denied the opportunity to exercise his right to withdraw from the gene transfer trial.

CONFLICT OF INTEREST

As noted above, any discussion about the adequacy of the informed consent dovetails with concerns about the researchers having a conflict of interest. Conflict of interest is a repeated theme throughout much of the research literature. Indeed, lack of consent and conflict of interest are the biggest challenges facing both researchers and research institutions.

After any adverse outcome, the claim is easily made that the conduct of the researchers was to aggrandize the research itself, that such was done at the expense of the well-being of the subject, and that the subject had not been fully informed about the potential for the adverse outcome. In such circumstances, it is easy to argue that appropriate informed consent was not provided because of the manifest conflict of interest.

In the Gelsinger case, there were deep-seated conflicts of interest. The principal researcher, the university itself, and less surprisingly, the sponsor, all had a significant financial interest in the therapy that was being tested on Jesse Gelsinger and the seventeen participants before him.[31] None of this was disclosed to Mr Gelsinger or to his family.[32]

In light of these alleged facts being established, it was not a long step to find that the researchers were in a conflict of interest. The question in the context of a negligence suit is whether such conflicts of interest need be disclosed. Whether on the test of 'full and frank' disclosure as defined in *Halushka*, or even on the less stringent material risk test enunciated in *Reibl*, it seems clear that conflicts of interest must be disclosed by researcher to gene therapy trial participants as part of the informed consent information they receive. The *Tri-Council Policy Statement*, as one example, stipulates that 'researchers or their qualified designated representatives shall provide prospective subjects with ... [information about] the presence of any apparent or actual or potential conflict of interest on the part of researchers, their institutions or sponsors.[33]

RESULTS FROM ANIMAL TRIALS

Regulations under the *Food and Drugs Act* now clearly lay out the stages or phases of clinical trials investigation. The phase of clinical trials immediately before trials on human subjects are those on animal subjects. The continuum is transparent and clearly demonstrates that in the appropriate circumstances, such as those noted in the Gelsinger case above, pertinent information about animal trials may need to be disclosed to human subjects.

To justify a gene transfer trial involving humans, most researchers would have to have garnered a considerable amount of evidence from animal trials. To then claim that such data are not relevant information in the informed consent process is both inconsistent and inappropriate. That is not to say that the failure to disclose all serious adverse events in animal trials establishes a breach of the standard of care owed to human subjects. Adverse events will be commonplace in many gene transfer trials. What must be disclosed is information about adverse events that is material, whether occurring in animal trials or human trials.

Causation

In order to establish a claim in negligence against a defendant or defendants, there must be a causal connection between the failure to meet the standard of care and the injuries suffered by the plaintiff. Stated otherwise, the injured party or those acting on his or her behalf must demonstrate that the injury flows from the breach of the standard of care.

Let us begin by assuming that the information with respect to certain animal trials discussed above should have been disclosed and was not disclosed. In order for the plaintiff to succeed, he or she would have to establish that the information withheld was so material that he or she would not have agreed to take part in the research if the information had been made available. The plaintiff must successfully argue that, 'but for the researchers' failure to disclose this information, I would not have participated in the research.'[34] Like the duty of care and standard of care elements, the burden for establishing causation lies on the plaintiff.[35] Depending upon the circumstance, this may pose a problem.

In the Gelsinger case, Jesse Gelsinger was not facing threat of death, or even decline, from his underlying medical condition, when he consented to participate in the gene transfer study. Although the defence case was not developed, it seems probable that a court would have held the failure to disclose material information as being causally linked to Mr Gelsinger's death; that is, had he known results of adenoviral transfer in the animal trials, he would not have agreed to participate in the research at all. The plaintiffs argued that the researchers' failure to disclose the true risk of the gene transfer caused Mr Gelsinger's participation. 'But for' that negligence, he would not have participated and would not have died.[36]

This may be contrasted to James Dent's situation. Mr Dent was undergoing a terminal process due to his underlying brain tumour. The defence would have tried to establish that Mr Dent, or another plaintiff with a like terminal condition, would have tried anything to combat the severity of their condition, including consenting to research, even where serious adverse events were expected. The argument would be that short of gene transfer offering a possible shot at a cure, death appeared imminent. In such circumstances, a court may well find that even with disclosure of the adverse events, Mr Dent would nonetheless have undergone the procedure. The 'but for' test is much harder to establish in the Dent case.[37]

The same is true with respect to the conflict of interest aspects of causation. In order to establish causation, plaintiffs must show, on a balance of probabilities, that they would have withheld consent had they been told, for example, of the financial interests in play. If the participant was cognizant of the possibility than his or her best interests could have been compromised by the conflict of interest, he or she might reasonably have withheld consent.

The decision by the Supreme Court of Canada in *Snell v. Farrell*[38] is significant to the question of onus in causation questions. Since *Snell*, it is clear that where the weight of the knowledge as to whether a certain act was the cause (or a material contribution) of a specific injury suffered by a layperson rests with the other party, such as a physician or researcher, the defence cannot simply sit back without calling evidence and then argue that the plaintiff has failed to establish causation. There is a very real risk that the court will find for the plaintiff in such a case.

For example, if there were two possible causes for the adverse outcome, only one of which relates to the conduct of the physician, the physician would be well advised to tender evidence to rebut the view that his or her conduct was the material cause of the outcome rather than simply hoping that the court will select the cause in which the physician or researcher was not involved.

In clinical trials, it is likely that the application of *Snell v. Farrell* will work to the benefit of plaintiffs. The balance of the knowledge about adverse events and about various interests engaged in the research trial is held by the sponsors, researchers, research institutions, and research ethics boards. When combined with (1) the higher standard for informed consent and disclosure in research activities, (2) the implications of conflict of interest, and (3) the burden of owing fiduciary duties to research participants, the court will likely look to the defendants to explain or refute an adverse outcome in an egregious fact situation. It is unlikely that the court will hold the plaintiff in such a circumstance to a strict burden of proof if troublesome aspects of the case are otherwise presented by the plaintiff.

Summary

It seems likely that the conduct complained of in both the Gelsinger and Dent cases amounted to a failure to provide adequate informed consent, for which the principal researchers responsible for the conduct of the gene therapy trial could have been found liable in negligence if the cases had gone to trial.

In order to guard against such a fate, researchers charged with the task of securing informed consent must disclose in a full and frank manner all material information, including potential serious adverse events. In addition, conflicts of interest must be disclosed and researchers, research institutions, and members of research ethics boards must exercise great caution in their professional duties. The burden of disclosure lies on the defendants. They must be candid and straightforward about the material risks and benefits of the research, and they must disclose clearly if there are any conflicts of interest about which they are aware.

III. Probable Defendants in a Lawsuit

In order to understand why various defendants may be named in a lawsuit, it is important to understand the litigation milieu in which legal proceedings are brought. For example, since the *Rules of Procedure* in Ontario[39] do not allow non-parties to be examined prior to a trial itself, except with leave of the court, the best strategy from a plaintiff's perspective is to 'name' everyone in the statement of claim. In this way, plaintiffs' counsel has a broad discretion to choose those whom he or she wishes to question about the incidents that gave rise to the harm from among the many players. Each defendant's potential liability will, however, play out differently. Defendants are only liable for those acts which they did or did not do in relation to the harm. While their actions may be thoroughly canvassed during preparation of the case, this does not mean that liability will be found against them, or even that they will be kept in the litigation to its conclusion.

Sponsors

As noted at the beginning of this chapter, the growth of gene transfer research has coincided with a maturation of the entire biotechnology sector. Gene transfer has enjoyed the support of industry-academia partnerships, while entire corporations have been set up to organize and finance gene transfer studies.

Sponsors of such research, typically the pharmaceutical manufacturer funding the study, have certain obligations.[40] These include ensuring that:

1. the clinical trial is scientifically sound and clearly described in the protocol;
2. the clinical trial is conducted in accordance with the protocol;
3. the quality assurance aspects of the protocol are implemented;
4. at each site, the clinical trial has secured approval of an REB;
5. medical care is given and medical decisions are made by a qualified investigator;
6. each individual involved in conducting the clinical trial is qualified by education, training, and experience;

7. written consent is obtained in accordance with governing laws and the protocol; and
8. records with respect to the clinical trials are kept and meet with regulatory standards regarding content, including all versions or amendments to the investigators' brochure, enrolment of participants, adverse events, and shipping of product or drug in question. The sponsor must also ensure retention of records for fifty years.

It is likely that any litigation will name the sponsors of the clinical trial or early therapy. Their involvement and obligations are too great and their pockets are too deep to be ignored by plaintiffs, regardless of their level of active participation in the clinical trial.[42]

Rsearchers/Investigators

Increasingly, plaintiffs are naming individual researchers as parties to the lawsuit. The researcher is the human face of the gene transfer trial and has the most direct contact with the patient. The responsibility for discharging the informed consent process lies not with the sponsor of the trial but with the researcher/investigator. Anger is often directed at the researcher and he or she is named in the proceedings along with the sponsor.

Under any negligence analysis, the first question to be asked is whether the researcher owes a duty of care to his or her subjects? The clear answer is 'yes.' In the *Halushka* case, the Saskatchewan Court of Appeal held two physician researchers and the University of Saskatchewan, at which the research took place, directly liable for trespass to the person and negligence during a research project in anaesthesia. More recently, the Quebec Superior Court in the *Weiss* case held researchers directly liable in a trial to test ophthalmic drops for controlling post-cataract surgery complications.

Whether the research is in the area of gene therapy or otherwise, there can be no doubt that the researchers owed Jesse Gelsinger and James Dent a duty of care. The relationship of researcher and subject is fiduciary in nature and carries with it a high burden of trust. Unlike a relationship between physician and patient alone, however, researchers may owe a number of different fiduciary duties, which may sometimes be in conflict with each other. For example, researchers owe fiduciary duties to the company sponsoring the gene therapy trial. Such a duty does not displace or take precedence over the duties owed to the research participants, but rather shows that researchers may face multiple fiduciary relationships. The situation gets more complex when the researcher is also the acting physician of the participant.[42] Nevertheless, it is clear law that a researcher owes a duty of care to the research participant or subject.

Whether the duty of care was breached will be a factually determined question. One must start, however, by determining the standard of care expected in the gene therapy trial and whether it was met. It may seem counter-intuitive to refer to a 'standard of care' in research cases where no immediate medical benefits are expected and where the gene therapy is not being used in a treatment capacity. If anything however, where the harm-to-benefit ratio is potentially so one-sided, the standard of care in medical research assumes a higher standard than that required for physician care. Some have suggested that it requires a 'gold standard.'[43]

Research Institutions

As governments have cut back on the amount of taxpayer money made available to support hospitals and universities, there has been a concerted effort on the part of these research institutions to utilize intellectual capital in fiscally rewarding ways. This has led to private-public partnerships aimed at developing concepts and ideas into tangible products. Hospitals and universities have been pursuing the commercial possibilities of gene therapy since research began.

It is likely, therefore, that hospitals and universities will be drawn into litigation either as the actual sponsor or as the entity between the sponsor and the researcher/investigator. In addition, the hospitals and universities often establish and take responsibility for the REB/IRBs.[44] Members of review boards are usually volunteers and often feel themselves over-stretched. They often have modest assets and no relevant insurance. Hospitals and universities can expect that they will be targeted as the deeper pocket behind the researcher/investigator and the members of REB/IRBs.[45]

Research Ethics Boards / Institutional Review Boards

Mechanisms have been developed to safeguard subject safety; two of the most important are the REB/IRBs and the investigator's brochure. Since the intent of both is to ensure the safety of those participating in clinical trials or early therapy, they will come under intense scrutiny in any subsequent litigation.

Depending upon the background to the litigation, a researcher/ investigator may try to limit his or her exposure by relying on the oversight role played by the research institution and the review board. This can, however, set up a contest among the named parties. For example, what happens if the researcher/investigator fails to report serious adverse events both to the participant and to the research institution or the review board? In the wake of the Gelsinger story, one report claimed that 94 per cent of serious adverse events occurring in the United States were not being reported to the appropriate authorities.[46]

Whether and for what reasons the research institution or the REB/ IRB will be found liable in such circumstances will depend on: (1) what they knew at the time; (2) what they should have known; and (3) the adequacy of the inquiry they undertook to determine what they should have known.

With the usual caveats, research institutes and review boards owe a duty of care to research participants. Institutions may be directly liable, as in *Weiss*, for failing to have certain equipment on hand.[47] Alternatively, they may be indirectly or vicariously liable where there is a relationship such as one of employment between the researcher and the research institution,[48] or between the review board and its members and the research institution. In *Weiss*, the research institute, a hospital, was found partially liable for the outcome due to the deficiencies in the conduct of the REB.

After the Gelsinger case, the U.S. Food and Drug Administration halted all gene therapy trials at the University of Pennsylvania because of what was alleged to be the institution's poor research oversight. It had already halted the work of the principal researcher.[49] Similarly, a recent decision by a State of Illinois Appellate Court noted that an IRB's failure to detect that consent forms had been inappropriately altered by the researcher, following IRB approval, amounted to a breach of its 'minimal duty' to follow up.[50] On its face, this decision seems to impose a standard of care that requires review boards to oversee all gene therapy trials continuously.[51]

The kind of 'minimal duty' described by the Illinois court is not yet common practice among review boards in either the United States or Canada. To date, there is no industry standard to guide the actions and governance of REB/IRBs. Moreover, the task of ongoing review is not straightforward. Even if a review board has adequate resources to monitor research, there is the question of whether they have access to the information necessary to do so effectively. The reporting of adverse events makes others a better point of responsibility in this regard than the board and its members.

Nonetheless, and despite the obvious difficulties facing review boards as a result of exposure to liability, it is likely that the law will evolve over the next few years to impose higher standards on them. After all, one might argue that ongoing monitoring is the very essence of review board, and that structures and policies should be put in place to secure effective ongoing reporting and follow up with clinical trials that have been approved by the board. This is particularly true with respect to REB/IRB obligations (1) to halt a trial with a material number of adverse events; (2) to disclose new information that may be material to the patients; and (3) to continue to have a duty to trial participants even after the trial itself is over.

The weight of liability is also likely to be attached to review boards with respect to conflict of interest matters. Both the Regulations under the *Food and Drugs Act* and the *Tri-Council Policy Statement* require conflicts to be monitored by review boards. The *Tri-Council Policy Statement* stipulates that all 'actual, perceived or potential conflicts of interest' must be made known to the boards,[52] while the new Regulations require them 'to ensure that conflict of interest situations are avoided and that the health and safety of trial subjects remain the paramount concern.'[53]

While these statements may sound laudable, in their present form review boards really do not have the ability to manage such conflicts of interest effectively. At least one court in the United States has raised this concern. The Maryland Court of Appeal has stated that IRBs are 'not designed, generally, to be sufficiently objective in the sense that they are as sufficiently concerned with the ethicality of the experiments they review as they are with the success of those experiments.'[54]

None of this is to excuse review boards or research institutions. Indeed, there is a high probability that the REB or IRB on the facts in either the Dent or Gelsinger cases would have been found liable for negligence with respect to overseeing the research trial.

Conclusion

It has often been said that the law lags behind science. While science pushes back brave new frontiers with the promise of a new day, the law 'sticks to its knitting.' In considering liability issues in the context of gene transfer research, the law will revert to a familiar analysis for breach of contract and tort of negligence. When discussing liability in the context of gene transfer research, the applicable legal framework is one that applies to all medical care, albeit with a higher standard to be met in research cases. Indeed, principles of informed consent and conflict of interest are by no means uniquely important for gene therapy trials.

Nonetheless, there are those who would quite rightly question whether the law in the area of research should be permitted to develop only as common law. The court may be unable to find the correct analogies when the evidence before it is at the cutting edge of science. The question then becomes whether, given that research with human subjects will be conducted, government should develop appropriate regulation to protect those participating as human subjects. Putting the onus on the human subjects to bring lawsuits based in negligence to remedy systemic wrongs is a heavy burden, even if individual claims against individual researchers and institutions are ultimately successful. Still, the law is likely to hold that an orderly evolution of case law, building on the insights of Justice Hall in the *Halushka* case, will best manage factual circumstances and claims that remain for the present as unimagined as the science that will give rise to them.

NOTES

The author is grateful to Matthew Herder for his contributions to the first draft of an earlier paper presented at the University of Toronto.

1 'Gene Therapy,' http://www.ornl.gov/TechResources/Human_Genome/medicine/genethera py.html.
2 As of the end of 2002, some forty gene therapy trials on humans have been undertaken in Canada. Fourteen were ongoing at the beginning of 2003, although none used retroviruses to insert the genes. The majority used adenoviruses, which are considered much safer. Scientists have warned that retroviruses can cause cancer because they permanently invade the DNA of the cells. See Brad Evenson, 'Toddler's Cancer Imperils Future of Gene Therapy: Virus Technique,' *National Post*, 16 January 2003.
3 Nine out of the eleven boys treated for X-SCID were essentially 'cured' by the treatment. They left hospital and began to lead normal, active lives.

4 Elliot Schiff, 'In the Service of Science,' CBC Television, *The National: The Magazine* (6 March 2000).

5 Only days before James Dent's death, a patient participating in an identical clinical trial in the United States had died. Dent was allegedly not informed of this death, despite having specifically asked to be kept informed of developments with respect to testing of the gene therapy. Both the Gelsinger and Dent trials passed research ethics boards; later criticism maintained that neither should have done so.

6 For an excellent and detailed discussion of the developing theories and case law in clinical research in the United States, see Sheila M. Brennan Connor and Karen D. McDonnell, 'Emerging Trends in Litigation Arising Out of Clinical Research' (paper presented at the Defence Research Institute conference held in New Orleans, 1–2 May 2003).

7 For an interesting discussion about whether traditional legal principles should apply to litigation in the context of clinical research, see E. Haavi Morreim, 'Litigation in Clinical Research: Malpractice Doctrines versus Research Realities' (2004) 32 J.L. Med. & Ethics 474. Dr Morreim argues that the courts have tended to categorize research injuries as a species of medical malpractice and have failed to recognize the difference between clinical trials and medical treatment. She argues that in applying traditional tort doctrines, the courts may leave research subjects without appropriate remedies and reciprocally, may subject investigators and sponsors to unfair standards of liability.

8 Kathleen Cranley Glass and Trudo Lemmens, 'Research Involving Humans,' in Jocelyn Downie, Timothy Caulfield, and Colleen Flood, eds., *Canadian Health Policy*, 2nd ed. (Markham, ON: Butterworths, 2002), 459 at 493.

9 Brennan Connor and McDonnell, 'Emerging Trends in Litigation Arising Out of Clinical Research.'

10 P.C. 2001-1042, C. Gaz. 2001.II.1116 at 1129.

11 Plaintiffs' counsel will often cite the *Nuremberg Code* and the *Declaration of Helsinki*, revised most recently in 2000 in Edinburgh, Scotland, as the basis upon which claims are advanced. Neither of these ethical statements, nor the *Tri-Council Policy Statement* (see note 13 below), has the force of law, but a number of the principles enunciated therein (particularly those dealing with informed consent and conflict of interest guidelines) have been embodied in case law which is directive to Canadian courts.

12 Medical Research Council of Canada, Natural Sciences and Engineering Research Council of Canada, Social Sciences and Humanities Research Council of Canada, *Tri-Council Policy Statement: Ethical Conduct for Research*

Involving Humans (Ottawa: Public Works and Government Services Canada, 1998).

13 There have been recent efforts in the United States to raise a new cause of action, variously known as 'dignity harm,' 'breach of duty to treat with dignity,' or 'breach of the right to be treated with dignity.' The thrust of this claim is that all humans deserve to be treated with an essential human dignity and that when research is conducted negligently, such dignity is offended. To date, the U.S. courts have been reluctant to expand such claims as new causes of action, preferring instead to rephrase them as part of the failure to provide adequate informed consent. See *Aderman v. Trustees of Univ. of Pa.*, No. 01-CV-6794(E.D. Pa. 2002), [2000] C.C.P. Philadelphia, Pa., No. 3285 ¶56–64 ; *Robertson v. McGee*, [2002] U.S. Dist. LEXIS 4072; *Abdullahi v. Pfizer, Inc.*, [2003] U.S. App. LEXIS 20704; *Afentakis v. Memorial Hospital*, 667 N.Y.S. 2d. 602 (Sup. Ct. 1997), as cited and discussed in Brennan Connor and McDonnell, 'Emerging Trends in Litigation Arising Out of Clnical Research' at 34–5.

14 [1980] 2 S.C.R. 880.

15 (1965) 53 D.L.R. (2d) 436 (Sask. C.A.).

16 Ibid. at ¶ 29 [emphasis added].

17 *Tri-Council Policy Statement* at Art. 2.4.

18 [1989] R.J.Q. 731 (Sup. Ct.).

19 Ibid. at headnote.

20 Glass and Lemmens, 'Research Involving Humans' at 495–6.

21 In Ontario, the scope of informed consent required in clinical practice is now detailed in s. 11 of the *Health Care Consent Act, 1996*, S.O. 1996, c. 2, Sched. A. It provides that the elements of informed consent include: (1) the consent must be related to the treatment; (2) the consent must be informed; (3) the consent must be given voluntarily; and (4) the consent must not be obtained through misrepresentation or fraud. In ensuring that the consent is 'informed,' the health practitioner must address (1) the nature of the treatment; (2) the expected benefits of the treatment; (3) the material risks of the treatment; (4) the material side effects of the treatment; (5) alternative courses of action; and (6) the likely consequences of not having the treatment. In addition, the health practitioner must provide responses to requests from the patients for any additional information.

22 See below for a more detailed discussion of concerns about researcher conflict of interest.

23 An informed consent form evidences that the discussion itself took place and can be supplemented with oral evidence from either plaintiff or defendant. In clinical trials and the transfer to gene therapy, the informed consent

information is quite detailed. Providing the form, however, is ancillary to, and not a substitute for, the necessary discussion with the subject or his legal representative.

24 Glass and Lemmens, 'Research Involving Humans' at 482.

25 Allegedly, the recruiters neglected to mention that the treatment could have a potentially toxic effect, and that monkeys injected with the genetically altered virus had become ill or died. See Alison Schneider, 'U. of Pennsylvania Settles Lawsuit Over Gene-Therapy Death,' *Chronicle of Higher Education* (6 November 2000).

26 Schiff, 'In the Service of Science.'

27 See note 5 above.

28 See below for further discussion. In *Hollis v. Dow Corning Corporation*, [1995] 4 S.C.R. 634, the Supreme Court of Canada held that a manufacturer has a duty to warn consumers of dangers inherent in a product's use about which it knew or ought to have known. The duty to disclose is a continuing one, requiring the manufacturer to warn not only of dangers known at the time of sale, but also discovered after the product has been sold and delivered. It is a logical extension to the duty to warn cases that a researcher who 'discovers' new or previously unappreciated risks or complications arising from ongoing research or early therapies has a duty to disclose such information expeditiously to participants in a study, and that a further consent process should be undertaken in light of this new information.

29 *Tri-Council Policy Statement* at Art. 2.1(a).

30 Ibid. at Art. 2.4(d).

31 Glass and Lemmens, 'Research Involving Humans' at 471.

32 Schneider, 'U. of Pennsylavnia Settles Lawsuit.'

33 *Tri-Council Policy Statement* at Art. 2.4(e).

34 Indeed, causation is often referred to as the 'but for' test.

35 See below, note 39.

36 Autopsy results have suggested that the adenovirus vector that was put directly into Jesse Gelsinger's hepatic artery appears to have triggered a massive immune response that led to his death. Eliot Marshall, 'Gene Therapy on Trial' (2000) 288 Science 951.

37 An autopsy report in the Dent case, delivered to Health Canada five months after the event, indicated that the drugs used in the second phase of the trial had contributed to his death. Nonetheless, the argument would still be presented that a reasonable person in Mr Dent's position would have continued with the therapy in light of his rather limited options. Schiff, 'In the Service of Science.'

38 [1990] 2 S.C.R. 311.

39 Rule 31.10, Rules of Civil Procedure, made under the *Courts of Justice Act*, R.R.O. 1990, Reg. 194 as amended.

40 While certain obligations exist at common law, these have been spelled out more recently in P.C. 2001-1042, c. Gaz. 2001. II. at subsection C.

41 The pharmaceutical industry has faced increasing pressure from both legislatures and editorial boards of medical journals to release more data about ongoing clinical drug trials. On 6 January 2005, the innovative pharmaceutical industry announced certain principles governing the disclosure of clinical trial information through publicly accessible clinical trial registries and databases. Under the voluntary proposals, details of ongoing clinical trials being performed to determine the therapeutic benefits of a clinical trial will be disclosed via free, publicly accessible databases regardless of outcome. The trial results will be published in a standard summary and will be available to patients and clinicians within one year of regulatory approval of a drug or, for post-approval trials, within one year of the trial being completed. For further information, see 'Joint Position on Disclosure of Clinical Trial Information via Clinical Trial Registries and Databases' released jointly on 6 January 2005 by the International Federation of Pharmaceutical Manufacturers and Associations (IFPMA), the European Federation of Pharmaceutical Industries and Associations (EFPIA), the Japanese Pharmaceutical Manufacturers Association (JPMA), and the Pharmaceutical Research and Manufacturers of America (PhRMA). See online: http://www.ifpma.org/News/NewsReleaseDetail.aspx?nID=2205.

42 A review of the duties and responsibilities existing between researcher and sponsor and between researcher and subject became the subject of scrutiny in a case at Toronto's Hospital for Sick Children involving Dr Nancy Olivieri and Apotex. The matters raised in that case are beyond the scope of this chapter. For a detailed review of the circumstances leading to the dispute and its aftermath, see Jon Thompson, Patricia Baird, and Jocelyn Downie, *The Olivieri Report* (Toronto: James Lorimer and Company, 2001).

43 Glass and Lemmens, 'Research Involving Humans' at 494–5.

44 Research Ethics Boards ('REBs') in Canada are known in the United States as Institutional Review Boards ('IRBs').

45 It is likely that hospitals and universities will be held vicariously liable for the activities of the REB unless there are clear contractual terms making them independent.

46 Schiff, 'In the Service of Science.'

47 Glass and Lemmens, 'Research Involving Humans' at 494.

48 Ibid.

49 Gretchen Vogel, 'FDA Moves against Penn Scientist' (2000) 290 Science 2049.
50 Glass and Lemmens, 'Research Involving Humans' at 497.
51 Continuous monitoring will be an almost overwhelming duty for most research institutions and their REBs and yet, the legal principles on which such a duty might be based are analogous to those of a manufacturer and its continuous duty to warn. See note 28 above.
52 *Tri-Council Policy Statement* at Art. 4.1. See also Glass and Lemmens, 'Research Involving Humans' at 472.
53 Glass and Lemmens, 'Research Involving Humans' at 472.
54 Ibid. at 475.

9 Legal Liability for Harm to Research Participants: The Case of Placebo-Controlled Trials

DUFF R. WARING AND KATHLEEN CRANLEY GLASS

Introduction

The choice of treatments for patients in the control arm of a randomized clinical trial (RCT or trial) has long been recognized as a contentious issue. Much has been written about the science and ethics of using placebo controls in RCTs when established, effective treatment is available.[1] However, little consideration has been given to questions of the legal liability of physician investigators if a research participant is harmed when effective treatment is withheld or withdrawn in the placebo arm of a trial.[2]

There is no Canadian or American legislation involving placebo-controlled trials, nor are we aware of a reported case in which damages have been awarded to a research participant for harm resulting from the use of placebos. How would a court decide such a case with relevant legal principles and available case law? This is a question with both legal and ethical implications. Our aim is to clarify the legal position by exploring two bases for the potential liability of physician investigators. First, we evaluate the administration of placebos 'through the lens of existing malpractice law.'[3] Second, we suggest that the enrolment of ill persons who seek established, effective treatment might constitute a separate claim for breach of fiduciary duty. We then look at defences and, in particular, the effect of an informed consent to assume any risks associated with being randomized to placebo in a clinical trial.

Our analysis is focused upon the potential for liability that arises when a fully informed research participant is harmed as a result of receiving placebo, and not therapy, in an RCT. The issue we wish to explore at this point is not the failure to adequately inform, but the failure to offer treatment in cases where there is an established, effective therapy. Subject to some special circumstances discussed below, the standard therapy would have been prescribed were the individuals not randomized to the placebo arm of a clinical trial. Problems associated with consent as a defence in such situations are considered later in the paper.

By enrolling in the clinical trial of a new therapeutic agent individuals are agreeing to bear some risk, since less will be known about the new therapy than about treatments that have already been studied. However, to initiate a trial, there must be sufficient pre-trial information (e.g., animal studies, tests on healthy volunteers, and/or case studies) to create genuine uncertainty among the expert clinical community about the comparative merits of each arm of the trial. This should amount to 'an honest, professional disagreement among expert clinicians about the preferred treatment' for a defined patient population. Freedman referred to this as a state of 'clinical equipoise' in which either arm of a clinical trial can be randomly offered as equivalent.[4] It recognizes that the normative evaluation of medical practice by way of law, regulation, or ethics occurs by reference to an expert community standard.[5] Freedman's notion of clinical equipoise thus provides a moral foundation for clinical trials in which the ethics of practice and research are combined.[6] In other words, people seeking treatment should not, by enrolling in a trial, be agreeing to medical attention that is known to be inferior to current clinical practice. With limited exceptions this forecloses the use of placebos when established, effective treatments exist.[7]

The ethical requirement that a trial proceed from a state of clinical equipoise can thus be seen as a fiduciary 'vehicle'[8] for evaluating the physician investigator's adherence to professional standards of patient-centred care. Since principles of civil liability apply to patient care and to biomedical research, we contend that a patient who is harmed by receiving a placebo could claim for damages against the physician investigator. While a patient may freely assume the risks of competently practised medical interventions, physicians cannot escape the professional duty to practise competent medicine by eliciting their patients' informed consent to do so.[9] This duty is premised on making the health of the patient the physician's first concern. We argue that this duty is not trumped by a competing interest in the advancement of research. Consequently, it also applies to physician investigators who enrol patients in RCTs.

Legal Framework for Compensating Harm to
Research Participants

While questions of criminal conduct could potentially arise in the context of research, we have limited our assessment to issues of civil legal liability.

Civil Liability for Medical Malpractice

Claims for medical malpractice are usually brought in the tort of negligence.[10] This cause of action requires the establishment of four elements: (1) the defendant must owe the plaintiff a duty of care; (2) the defendant must breach the legally established standard of care; (3) the plaintiff must suffer loss or injury; and (4) the defendant's conduct must have been the actual and legal cause of the plaintiff's injury.[11] Medical malpractice is thus a legal fault arising from a physician's failure to provide the required standard of care.

American case law has expressed a reasonable care standard as a legally enforceable, non-delegable duty of physicians to render professional services. These services must be consistent with the objectively ascertained, minimally acceptable level of competence that physicians can be expected to apply given their qualifications, expertise, and the circumstances of the case. In sum, the physician's duty of care is to treat each patient 'with such reasonable diligence, skill, competence, and prudence as are practiced by minimally competent physicians in the same specialty or general field of practice throughout the United States, who have available to them the same general facilities, services, equipment and options.'[12]

In Canada, a physician who treats a patient must use 'a reasonable degree of skill and knowledge and must exercise a reasonable degree of care,' meeting the standard of the 'normal, prudent practitioner of the same experience and standing.'[13] The test of whether a physician meets this standard is an objective one. The provision of care is measured against a reasonable physician who possesses and exercises the skill, knowledge, and judgment of the normal, prudent practitioner of his or her special group. In making this comparison, reference is made to the particular circumstances at the material time.[14] The standard of care is influenced by the foreseeable risk: the greater the risk, the higher the standard of care. The highest standard of care is expected of a physician using a new or experimental procedure or treatment.[15] There is thus 'an increased and extended duty of care' to the research participant.[16]

ANALYSIS

As noted above, there is no case law directly on point for placebo-controlled trials. However, using an analysis based on common law principles of legal liability and the few relevant American and Canadian non-placebo research cases, we believe that a research participant who is harmed by the denial of established effective treatment in the placebo arm of a trial might have an action in malpractice against the physician investigator. The four elements of the action might be established with the following arguments.

1 *The defendant owes the plaintiff a duty of care.* In the context of research, did the physician investigator and patient participant have a 'doctor-patient' relationship? In other words, did the physician 'hold out' the ability and willingness to treat, diagnose, and refer patients?[17] Ordinarily, potential research participants are approached as patients when they are seeking medical assistance in hospitals, clinics, or private physicians' offices.

Legal commentary holds that a physician investigator's main concern should be the health and well-being of research participants.[18] Physicians themselves recognize the existence of a doctor-patient relationship with research participants. The priority of this concern is reflected in international and professional guidelines for ethical conduct in biomedical research. The Preamble to the World Medical Association's *Declaration of Helsinki* recognizes the doctor-patient relationship with the phrase '[t]he health of my patient will be my first consideration.' It states further that 'considerations related to the well-being of the human subject should take precedence over the interests of science and society.' Hence it is the duty of physician investigators to 'protect the life, health, privacy, and dignity of the human subject.'[19]

The American Medical Association (AMA) *Current Opinions* on its *Code of Medical Ethics* states that 'in a clinical investigation primarily for treatment,' the physician should evince the same concern for the welfare, safety, and comfort of the research participant as is required of a physician who provides medical care to a patient outside of any clinical investigation. Indeed, in research designed to test the efficacy of treatment, the physician investigator 'must recognize that the patient-physician relationship exists and that professional judgment and skill must be exercised in the best interest of the patient.'[20]

Miller and Brody have suggested that the traditional obligations of doctors to patients do not apply to biomedical research. In their view, physician investigators are involved in a different enterprise from physicians in clinical practice. The former have an obligation to answer 'clinically relevant questions,' while the latter must provide 'optimal patient care.' The different obligation of physician investigators allegedly releases them from the duty of care that applies to physicians in clinical practice. Miller and Brody argue that the relationship between physician investigators and research participants should be judged differently, that is, investigators only have a duty to avoid exploiting research participants by exposing them to excessive risk.[21]

However, the weight of legal evidence goes against their arguments. Physician investigators have never been granted legal immunity from the obligations of clinical care. In most major jurisdictions, the general rules of medical law are equally applicable to experimental procedures, whether carried out with a therapeutic purpose or not.[22] There is no separate regime of liability for medical research with human participants.[23] While the standard of care may be different for research and for therapy, as discussed below, we have found nothing in either U.S. or Canadian case law to indicate that an injured participant could not seek compensation in negligence in the same way a patient could.

2 *The defendant breached the established standard of care.* Once it has been established that the physician-investigator has a doctor-patient relationship with the research participant, and owes a duty of care, we must define the standard by which the defendant will be judged. International commentary establishes a standard of care for physician investigators in biomedical research. Although research and therapy can be distinguished, they often occur together, as when research is designed to evaluate a particular therapeutic intervention involving patients who suffer from the illness the therapy is designed to treat.[23] Giesen concludes that the standard of care imposed on physicians in the context of therapeutic practice 'will be unchanged' for physician investigators who combine research and therapy in RCTs. It is only their expected level of skill and care and the measures for ensuring the informed consent of research participants 'that will vary in proportion to the element of novelty and the presence of a research purpose.'[24] According to Canadian case law, 'the highest standard of care is expected of the doctor using a new or experimental procedure or treatment.'[25] A recent decision of the Quebec Court of Appeal[26] clearly confirms that when research in medical centres involves clinical procedures, research participants can rightly expect that the interventions

they undergo will be judged by the standard of care that physicians owe to their patients.[27]

As noted above, the AMA's *Code of Ethics* and the *Declaration of Helsinki* place the health of patient participants above the interests of science and society. Both the code and declaration might be admissible as legal evidence of the required standard of care in appropriate cases.[28] While not authority for American or Canadian courts, it is interesting to note that the German Federal Constitutional Court has addressed the relationship between medical ethics and law: 'Professional medical ethics do not stand separate from the law ... What the rules of medical ethics demand of a physician, will at the same time and to a large extent also be the legal obligation that has to be fulfilled. It is in the medical professional field much more than in any other social relationship ... that ethical considerations are inextricably linked with considerations of a legal nature.'[29] These non-legal guidelines, codes, or policy statements might assist a plaintiff in applying general rules of medical law to research with human participants. They might be especially important in judicial proceedings when the law is unclear.[30]

They were relevant, for instance, in the U.S. decision of *Grimes v. Kennedy Krieger Institute*.[31] This case involved non-therapeutic, potentially harmful research with children. The Court of Appeals of Maryland noted the paucity of judicial decisions involving human research participants and the consequent difficulty of developing a '"common law" of human experimentation.' It held that this 'absence of judicial precedent' makes documents like the *Nuremberg Code* 'all the more important.' In determining the applicable legal duties, the majority was clear: 'We are guided ... by these international "codes" or "declarations,"' as well as by government studies and 'other writings.'[32]

The court held that 'the breach of obligations imposed on researchers by the *Nuremberg Code*, might well support actions in negligence ...'[33] Indeed, non-therapeutic research that does not prioritize the welfare of the child participant over the interests of science and society[34] raised 'serious questions' under both the *Nuremberg Code* and the *Declaration of Helsinki*.[35] The court affirmed that its 'policy considerations' against permitting children to be exposed to potential harm, even with parental substitute consent, were guided by the *Nuremberg Code*.[36] The court also considered the *Declaration of Helsinki* in its assessment of the ethical appropriateness of the research.[37]

The *Nuremberg* and *Helsinki* documents referenced by the court embody principles protecting research participants that had been the subject of public and professional support since the 1940s and 1960s respectively. While such extra-legal documents might be no less relevant when research and therapy are combined, their interpretation is subject to ongoing debate. Current controversy relates to recent amendments to the *Helsinki* document in the context of placebo-controlled trials, because they derogate from the original principles of upholding participants' interests over the interests of science and society. We think that this debate is sufficient to warn researchers, Research Ethics Boards – Institutional Review Boards, and the judiciary against relying on the current version of this document relating to placebo as if it set binding standards on research.[38]

Legal principle supports the claim that physician investigators must meet the standard of care of the 'normal prudent practitioner of the same experience and standing,'[39] if not a 'heightened standard of care' for a novel treatment.[40] Randomizing patients to the placebo arm of a trial prevents them from receiving either established therapy or a novel therapy that is thought by many in the expert clinical community to be equivalent. Would this be considered an action below the standard of care? We need to ask, '[w]ould a normal, prudent practitioner have offered an effective treatment to a patient with this condition?' We acknowledge that some competent patients might be altruistic enough to refuse treatment for a minor condition to participate in research 'when withholding such therapy will not lead to undue suffering or the possibility of irreversible harm of any magnitude.'[41] Unless there are other special circumstances (e.g., where no proven effective treatment exists, where a patient is unresponsive to such treatment, where a patient has previously rejected established treatment because of negative side effects, when established treatment has been called into question by new evidence warranting doubt concerning its presumed net therapeutic advantage, or when the trial is for an 'add on' therapy in which all patients receive standard treatment plus placebo),[42] we suggest that replacing effective treatment with placebo controls would constitute negligence. Given the above, the notion that physician investigators are absolved from the obligations of physicians who only provide clinical care has no legal foundation.

3. The breach resulted in harm. Civil liability of the physician investigator for giving placebos in RCTs depends on whether the patient has suffered damage and whether it can be proven that an appropriate intervention, whether a pharmacologically active substance, or a diagnostic or surgical intervention, 'would have produced better effects.'[43] Without a centralized system for reporting adverse events, it is difficult to generalize about the effects of placebo-controlled trials. Examples of potential harm in such trials have been studied most thoroughly in psychiatry. This is particularly important given the large number of placebo-controlled trials in this area.

Recent research into the withdrawal of neuroleptics suggests serious clinical risk to patients whose medications are abruptly withdrawn in placebo-controlled drug trials. Gilbert et al. found uncommon risks of serious adverse effects such as hematemesis, neuroleptic malignant syndrome, emergent dyskinesia, tardive akathisia, and progressive Parkinsonism.[44]

Viguera and Baldessarini et al. conducted a study involving 1,210 schizophrenic patients, most of whom were participants in the placebo arms of RCTs from 1969 to 1995. They compared continued versus discontinued antipsychotic treatment and concluded that there is a high early risk of psychotic morbidity after the abrupt withdrawal of oral neuroleptics:[45] 'Appreciable increases in relapses can be detected even within days of discontinuation of medication in some particularly vulnerable or treatment-sensitive persons.'[46]

Although Gilbert et al. noted that patients who deteriorated after neuroleptic withdrawal often recompensated quickly when treatment was resumed,[47] some evidence suggests that others 'may have a difficult time returning to their previous level of function.' Abrupt withdrawal may actually worsen the patient's condition by contributing to 'treatment nonresponsiveness.'[48] The clinical risks of morbidity might occasionally exceed those associated with the natural history of the untreated illness. There is a 'distinct probability' that schizophrenia becomes more difficult to treat with each relapse.[49] Drawing on studies of both schizophrenia and depression, Baldessarini and Viguera claim that 'worsening of primary disorders often follows the rapid removal of long-term psychotropic treatment.'[50] Thus the withdrawal of medication required for randomization in a placebo-controlled trial may worsen some patients' conditions, that is, it may make them more difficult to treat after medication is resumed. If so, the resulting harm may not be limited to the symptoms endured during the trial. Those symptoms can be harmful enough, although proponents of placebo-controlled trials often overlook them.

Symptoms that might be expected for participants in the placebo arm of an anti-psychotic drug trial might include increased paranoia, delusions, profoundly confused thinking, agitation, impaired self-care, and increased risk of aggressive behaviour and harm to others.[51] These are the direct harms of schizophrenia that initially lead patients to seek treatment. There can be painful consequences to this 'clinical turmoil,' including increased risk of legal confinement 'with attendant psycho-social and financial costs, increased risk of suicide, and severe disruption of the lives of the patient and family.'[52]

There is anecdotal evidence that details such as relapse rates have been kept out of the informed consent process because they were 'overly frightening.' Put another way, such details might discourage enrolment in RCTs. The altruism that supposedly motivates some psychiatric patients to enrol in placebo-controlled trials may not endure an understanding of the potential for adverse effects. The following remark by a consumer who has considered this issue should not be ignored: 'Do you think people say, "Gee, I'll sign up for more suffering?" Many of us suffer enough on our own.'[53]

There is suggestive evidence that slow, tapered discontinuation might limit or delay relapse in schizophrenia. An emerging opinion is that a slow taper over a period of weeks or months is clinically recommended.[54] Even so, there is no evidence that a slow taper followed by a placebo will prevent relapse in patients who responded favourably to standard anti-psychotics before enrolling in the trial. As for newly diagnosed patients, there is no precedent in the current clinical management of schizophrenia or depression for exacerbating a patient's condition by substituting placebos for effective treatment. Even if there are patients whom physicians would leave temporarily untreated, random assignment to treatment versus placebo is unknown in clinical care.

While definitions of schizophrenic relapse vary, they usually involve clinical assessment or the use of rating scales scores 'to indicate the worsening of psychotic symptoms severe enough to warrant hospitalization or reinstitution of antipsychotic treatment.'[55] If a patient participant must prove injury in a negligence action, then exacerbation of the psychotic symptoms that initially required treatment should constitute direct harm. Some have claimed that the import of this harm can be minimized in the interests of science. It has been suggested that there is 'negligible evidence for any lasting disadvantage even in the face of substantial contemporaneous symptomatic disadvantage.'[56] Second, it has been noted that risk is limited to the time the participant is enrolled in the trial.[57] We fail to see how substantial symptomatic disadvantage, let alone relapse, is rendered acceptable if it is so limited. These arguments might limit the quantum of damages in a negligence action, but they would not obviate the suffering on which the plaintiff's claim is based.

Similar concerns might be raised about antidepressant drug trials that use placebo controls. Geddes et al. pooled data from thirty-one placebo-controlled, randomized trials involving 4,410 participants who had responded favourably to antidepressants. The aim of the study was to determine whether continuing treatment with antidepressants reduces the risk of relapse (i.e., the return of symptoms during a period of remission) or recurrence (i.e., a new episode during a period of recovery) of depressive symptoms. The authors concluded that continued antidepressant therapy for at least another year would benefit many patients who remain at appreciable risk of recurrence after four to six months. This continued treatment could reduce the risk of relapse by 70 per cent, as opposed to treatment discontinuation. They noted, however, that the average rate of relapse on placebo was 41 per cent compared to 18 per cent on active treatment.[58]

Nor are the problems of clinical disadvantage from delayed treatment or use of placebo limited to psychiatry: 'Evidence exists that delay or modification of treatment may modify the long-term course of illness on chronic diseases such as hypertension and rheumatoid arthritis. For these diseases, a period of poor disease control may result in long-term, irreversible organ damage.'[59]

4 *The defendant's conduct was the actual and legal cause of that injury.* After proving the standard of care, its breach, and a resulting injury, the plaintiff must prove a causal link between the defendant's negligence and the injury.[60] The plaintiff must prove on a balance of probabilities that, but for the defendant's tortious conduct, the plaintiff would not have sustained the injury complained of.[61] The defendant's conduct must be both the factual cause and the proximate cause of the injury. Determining the factual cause requires an inquiry into the cause-and-effect relationship that brought about the injury.[62]

Our analysis of causation parallels that of Mary Thomson in the previous chapter. According to the Supreme Court of Canada in *Snell v. Farrell*, this 'substantial connection' need not be determined with 'scientific precision.' A lesser standard is required by law.[63] The issue of whether a substantial causal link can be determined is a practical question of fact which is best inferred by 'ordinary common sense.' Indeed, when facts lie particularly within the defendant's knowledge, 'very little affirmative evidence' from the plaintiff will justify an inference of causation in the absence of evidence to the contrary. Although the defendant risks an adverse inference of liability in the absence of evidence to the contrary, this does not shift the burden of proof to the defendant. Rather, the defendant can assume a 'provisional or tactical burden' which allows the introduction of evidence in an attempt to rebut the plaintiffs claim.[64] If such evidence is adduced by the defendant, then the trial judge can weigh it in 'a robust and pragmatic approach to the facts' that can 'enable an inference of negligence to be drawn even though medical or scientific expertise cannot arrive at a definitive conclusion.'[65]

This pragmatic approach, which distinguishes between the respective functions of the trier of fact and the expert witness, is reflected in U.S. jurisprudence. The U.S. Supreme Court has held that a jury's power to draw an inference that the defendant's medical negligence caused the plaintiff's injury cannot be impaired 'by the failure of any medical witness to testify that it was in fact the cause.' Neither can it be impaired 'by the lack of medical unanimity as to the respective likelihood of the potential causes of the aggravation [injury] or by the fact that other potential causes of the aggravation existed and were not conclusively negatived by the proofs.'[66]

Determining the proximate cause requires the court to find that the injury sustained was foreseeable to a reasonable person in the defendant's position. This test of foreseeability is flexibly applied. To some extent, defendants in general negligence law take their victims as they find them. Picard and Robertson cite the following policy reasons against a strict application of this foreseeability test: 'the difficulty of determining with certainty what is foreseeable, the protection of vulnerable persons, the deterrence of substandard conduct, and the wider distribution of loss due to tortious activity.'[67] According to Linden on tort law, if the defendant's negligence renders the plaintiff's skull thin, that is, makes the plaintiff more susceptible to additional injury or sickness, then 'the defendant is responsible for the further complications.'[68]

In order to meet the burden of proof, a plaintiff would need to marshall evidence of the type described above for the treatment of patients with schizophrenia or rheumatoid arthritis that failure to treat, or delay in treatment resulting from randomization to the placebo arm of a clinical trial, exacerbated symptoms or caused permanent damage.

Breach of Fiduciary Duty

The physician-patient relationship is often described as fiduciary, that is, a relationship of utmost good faith. 'The law defines a fiduciary as a person entrusted with power or property to be used for the benefit of another and legally held to the highest standard of conduct.'[69] As fiduciaries, physicians must act in the best interests of their patients and must not allow their own interests to conflict with them.[70]

How useful is the notion of fiduciary duty in the context of American and Canadian law relating to medical treatment? Although breach of fiduciary duty can give rise to an alternative cause of action against a physician,[71] this action has limited scope. In U.S. case law, the specific purposes for which fiduciary principles have been applied to physicians include requiring them to (a) not abandon patients; (b) keep patient information confidential; (c) obtain informed consent to treatment; and (d) disclose to patients any financial interest in clinical research.[72] Rodwin concludes that, apart from these circumstances, physicians in clinical practice 'are not held to fiduciary standards, especially with respect to financial conflicts of interest.' There is thus a gap between the practice of some U.S. physicians and the 'fiduciary ideal.'[73]

By contrast, Canadian courts, particularly the Supreme Court of Canada, 'have begun to show renewed interest in the fiduciary aspects of medical practice. It is likely that the principles of fiduciary law will have a significant impact on the rights of patients and the potential liability of doctors.'[74] While Canadian case law also applies fiduciary principles in limited circumstances, the Supreme Court of Canada has held that a physician has a fiduciary duty 'to make a proper disclosure of information to the patient.'[75] Physicians who have sexually abused their patients have also been held liable in damages for breaching their fiduciary duty.[76]

How might a physician investigator breach fiduciary duties in an RCT? Allowing ill patient participants to deteriorate in a placebo arm might amount to a subordination of their health in favour of scientific or financial interests. The Supreme Court of California[77] has determined that an interest in research can conflict with an interest in the patient participant's health. The U.S. court held that a physician investigator's eagerness to promote the advancement of science may result in riskier experimental treatments. The physician investigator must disclose to a participant 'any personal interests unrelated to the patient's health, whether research or economic, that may affect the physician's professional judgement.' An action for conversion was dismissed even though the physician converted the patient participant's blood products into a marketable commodity without consent. But the action for breach of the fiduciary duty to disclose financial interests in the research was accepted.[78]

Breach of fiduciary duty may become an important cause of action for injury in placebo-controlled trials because malpractice law generally ignores financial conflicts of interest. Physicians may receive financial benefits well beyond remuneration for professional services if they recruit patient participants or conduct trials. They may also have a financial relationship with the sponsor of the trial. Professional rewards, such as publications, promotion, and reputation in the research community are often competing interests.[79] These interests create the potential for an investigator's conflict with the primary duty of care to the patient. An RCT with a placebo arm is not designed to benefit patients in that trial. It is designed for the benefit of others, whether they are future patients, investigators, sponsors, or investors. Patients injured from lack of treatment in the placebo arm may have an action for breach of fiduciary duty when other interests are put above their well-being.

Studies examining the role of trust in patients' decisions to participate in research show that patients trusted their physicians to never endorse options that were not in their best interests.[80] This demonstrates the importance of physician investigators' fiduciary duty in RCTs, and their obligation to maintain it.

The Nature of Professional Obligations

Whether looking at negligence and the duty of care or breach of fiduciary duty, we find that the law does not allow physicians to 'opt out' of their professional obligations when conducting research. Even with the patient's informed consent, physician investigators have no professional or legal mandate to prescribe substandard treatments. It is generally not open to the doctor and patient to bargain away the 'guaranteed' level of professional competence: '[T]he very existence of tort law represents an element of paternalism in the law: we do not allow people unlimited discretion to choose what medical treatment they wish. The law protects them from making "poor" choices, on the theory that people are vulnerable to making such choices when it comes to health matters.'[81]

This reasoning can be applied to patients who choose to enrol in RCTs and consent to the chance of receiving placebos in lieu of effective treatment. Courts could be expected 'to take a very hard look at the use of placebo controls in cases where effective standard treatment exists, and to find that an investigator enrolling sick patients who may be assigned to placebo has, by definition, fallen below the existing standard of clinical practice.'[82]

The Defence of Informed Consent

There are potential defences available to physician investigators. Chief among them is an appeal to the patient's liberty in choosing to participate in a placebo-controlled trial. Both law and medicine put a high premium on individual autonomy. Some may argue that if patients are competent, well informed, and autonomous, then the choice to participate should always be theirs.[83] When coupled with informed consent, the notion of allowing altruistic patient participants to assume risk for the benefit of future persons has a certain appeal. Thus a defendant might argue that an informed, mentally capable participant voluntarily assumed the risk of receiving a placebo when consenting to enter the trial.

There are numerous arguments against this appeal to liberty. While the law allows for a defence of voluntary assumption of risk, the circumstances for its use are very limited. Some jurisdictions prohibit the waiver of liability for negligent infliction of bodily harm.[84] Further, a defendant cannot use such an agreement 'to escape responsibility for the consequences of his negligence,' unless it has been made unequivocally clear what is being waived, 'as by using the word "negligence" itself' in the agreement or consent form.[85] When has the process for obtaining informed consent, let alone a consent form, ever specified that the administration of placebos is substandard treatment that could otherwise ground a malpractice claim?

There are public policy considerations concerning the safety of research participants and the practice of medicine that weigh against unreasonable assumptions of risk. Indeed, courts have refused to uphold agreements that purport to waive liability for negligence 'where one party is at such obvious disadvantage in bargaining power that the effect of the contract is to put him at the mercy of the other's negligence.'[86] Again, tort law does not allow people unlimited discretion in their choice of medical treatment.[87] Moreover, it is a recognized principle of tort law that if plaintiffs surrender their better judgment 'upon an assurance that the situation is safe, or that it will be remedied, or on a promise of protection,' then they do not assume any risk. An exception would be a case in which 'the danger is so obvious and so extreme that there can be no reasonable reliance upon the assurance.'[88] Yet no one is suggesting that placebo-controlled trials be undertaken in cases of extreme risk. Nor is there a rationale for calling negligible risk an issue of malpractice. The focus of concern is on risks that fall between those that are extreme and those that are negligible.

As a matter of public policy, allowing patients to waive their physicians' professional standards of care will arguably have an adverse impact upon the practice of medicine and public health. Further, the notion that patient participants should fully understand the choices they are making to enter a trial is an ideal that is not always met. Randomization is a difficult concept for many to grasp. Studies have shown that many patient participants do not believe that they are allocated by chance to the arms in a trial. Many believe that they are allocated on the basis of their individual therapeutic needs.[89]

In short, the appeal to liberty fails on both practical and theoretical grounds. Every major code of ethics since the *Nuremberg Code* has recognized that adequate participant consent *and* an acceptable risk/benefit ratio are two independent preconditions for clinical research. As independent and necessary preconditions, issues of consent and of risk/benefit must each be resolved satisfactorily before a trial can proceed.[90]

Arguments on the limitations of consent might be sufficient to refute a defence based on the voluntary, informed assumption of risk. But even the most fully informed and capable consent should not justify substandard clinical practices in medical research. We argue that research participants 'cannot consent to otherwise unethical research ... If autonomous choice were all that mattered, there would be no need for an interdisciplinary debate [in a research ethics board] about the particular merits, benefits and risks of a study.'[91]

The U.S. Court of Appeals in the *Grimes* case affirmed the tenet that a participant's consent to research is not a reliable indication that the research is justified. Nor is consent the sole justificatory consideration. In sum, 'researchers cannot ever be permitted to immunize themselves completely by reliance on consents ... A researcher's duty is not created by, or extinguished by, the consent of a research subject or by IRB [Institutional Review Board] approval.'[92] That court noted that in consumer and contract law, respect for consensual arrangements is often balanced against other concerns. This can result in the substitution of the supposedly better judgment of the legislature or the judiciary about what is really in a person's best interest.[93] The Supreme Court of Canada has held that 'the fact that a patient acquiesces or agrees to a form of treatment does not absolve a physician of his or her duty if the treatment is not in accordance with medical standards.'[94] The goals of human health that motivate research into novel therapies ought to be reflected in a higher moral standard than the *caveat emptor* of the marketplace.[95]

Conclusion

There are no judgments or statutes offering specific guidance concerning the use of placebos as a control in randomized clinical trials. We believe that the arguments made above, based on legal principles and cases involving non-placebo medical research, may be persuasive in circumstances where a participant is harmed when established, effective therapy is withheld or withdrawn in the placebo arm of a trial. Voluntary assumption of risk through informed consent may not be sufficient to justify a breach of fiduciary duty or the practice of what would ordinarily be considered substandard medicine. Participants and investigators, as well as their institutions, sponsors, and government regulators, should be aware that those harmed in this way may have legal recourse.

NOTES

Duff Waring would like to acknowledge Genome Canada through the Ontario Genomics Institute and the Stem Cell Genomics and Therapeutics Network through the Natural Sciences and Engineering Resource Council for their generous support during the preparation of this chapter. Kathleen Glass's work on this chapter was funded by the Canadian Institutes of Health Research and the Social Sciences and Humanities Council of Canada.

 1 Henry K. Beecher, 'Surgery as Placebo: A Quantitative Study of Bias' (1961) 176 J. Am. Med. Assoc. 1102; Robert Temple, 'Government Viewpoint of Clinical Trials' (1982) 16 Drug Information Journal 10; Benjamin Freedman, 'Placebo-Controlled Trials and the Logic of Clinical Purpose' (1990) 12:6

IRB: A Review of Human Subjects Research 1; Kenneth J. Rothman and Karin B. Michels, 'The Continuing Unethical Use of Placebo Controls' (1994) 331 New Eng. J. Med. 394; Robert Temple, 'Problems in Interpreting Active Control Equivalence Trials' (1996) 4 Accountability in Research 267; and Robert Temple and Susan S. Ellenberg, 'Placebo-Controlled Trials and Active Control Trials in the Evaluation of New Treatments: Part 1: Ethical and Scientific Issues' (2001) 133 Annals Internal Med. 455.

2 See, however, prior works by the authors: Benjamin Freedman, Kathleen Cranley Glass, and Charles Weijer, 'Placebo Orthodoxy in Clinical Research II: Ethical, Legal, and Regulatory Myths' (1996) 24 J. L. Med. & Ethics 252 at 256; Kathleen Cranley Glass and Duff Waring, 'Effective Trial Design Need Not Conflict with Good Patient Care' (2002) 2:2 Am. J. Bioethics 25 at 26; Kathleen Cranley Glass and Duff Waring, 'The Physician/Investigator Obligation to Patients Participating in Research: The Case of Placebo-Controlled Trials' (2005) 33:3 J. Law Med. & Ethics 375–85.

3 Michelle Oberman, 'Mothers and Doctor's Orders: Unmasking the Doctor's Fiduciary Role in Maternal-Fetal Conflicts' (2000) 94 Nw. U.L. Rev. 451 at 459.

4 Benjamin Freedman, 'Equipoise and the Ethics of Clinical Research' (1987) 317 New Eng. J. Med. 141 at 144.

5 Ibid.; 'Ethics and Placebo-Controlled Thrombolytic Trials: The Future' (1991) 2 Coronary Artery Disease 849 at 850.

6 Charles Weijer, 'When Argument Fails' (2002) 2:2 American Journal of Bioethics 10.

7 Freedman, Glass, and Weijer, 'Placebo Orthodoxy II' at 253.

8 Oberman, 'Mothers and Doctor's Orders' at 459.

9 Freedman, Glass, and Weijer, 'Placebo Orthodoxy II' at 254.

10 Dan B. Dobbs, The Law of Torts, vol. 1 (St Paul, MN: West Publishing, 2001) at 269; Gerald Robertson, 'Negligence and Malpractice,' in Jocelyn Downie, Timothy Caulfield, and Colleen Flood, eds., Canadian Health Law and Policy, 2d ed. (Markham, ON: Butterworths, 2002) 91; Michael A. Jones, Medical Negligence (London: Sweet and Maxwell, 1991) at 20. See also Dieter Giesen, International Medical Malpractice Law: A Comparative Law Study of Civil Liability Arising from Medical Care (Dordrecht: Nijhoff, 1988) at ¶ 30–1; and Joseph H. King, Jr, The Law of Medical Malpractice in a Nutshell, 2d ed. (St Paul, MI: West Publishing, 1986) at 9.

11 Dobbs, Law of Torts at 631; Robertson, 'Negligence and Malpractice' at 91; Ellen I. Picard and Gerald B. Robertson, Legal Liability of Doctors and Hospitals in Canada, 3rd ed. (Toronto: Carswell, 1996) at 174. See also King, Law of Medical Malpractice at 9; Marcia Mobilia Boumil and Clifford Elias, The Law

of Medical Liability in a Nutshell (St Paul, MN: West Publishing 1995) at 24;
John G. Fleming, *The Law of Torts*, 8th ed. (Sydney: Law Book, 1992) at 102–3.

12 See *Hall v. Hilbun*, 466 So.2d 856 at 858 (Miss. 1985).

13 *Crits and Crits v. Sylvester* (1956), 1 D.L.R. (2d) 502 at 508 (Ont. C.A.), aff'd
[1956] S.C.R. 991.

14 Picard and Robertson, *Legal Liability of Doctors and Hospitals* at 186.

15 Ibid. at 193, 195.

16 Dieter Giesen, 'Civil Liability of Physicians for New Methods of Treatment
and Experimentation: A Comparative Examination' (1995) 3 Med. L. Rev.
22 at 30.

17 Picard and Robertson, *Legal Liability of Doctors and Hospitals* at 1–8.

18 Giesen, 'Civil Liability of Physicians' at 29: 'The interest of the sick person
in receiving therapeutic treatment, where this is most conducive to his
recovery, always takes precedence over the interests of science and medical
progress.' See also Giesen, *International Medical Malpractice Law* at ¶ 1200.

19 *Declaration of Helsinki*, 18th World Medical Association General Assembly,
June 1964 (amended October 1975, October 1983, September 1989, October
1996, October 2000), Arts. 3, 5, 10, 15. See also Medical Research Council of
Canada, Natural Sciences and Engineering Research Council of Canada &
Social Sciences and Humanities Research Council of Canada, *Tri-Council
Policy Statement: Ethical Conduct for Research Involving Humans* (Ottawa:
Public Works and Government Services Canada, 1998) at i.4.

20 American Medical Association Council on Ethical and Judicial Affairs, *Code
of Medical Ethics* (Chicago: American Medical Association Press, 2004–5) at
Art. E-2.07, Clinical Investigation, http:// www.ama-assn.org/ama/pub/
category/2498.html. See also ibid. at Art. E-2.075, The Use of Placebo Controls in Clinical Trials, which states: 'In general, the more severe the consequences and symptoms of the illness under study, the more difficult it will
be to justify the use of a placebo control when alternative therapy exists.
Consequently, there will almost certainly be conditions for which placebo
controls cannot be justified.'

21 Franklin G. Miller and Howard Brody, 'What Makes Placebo-Controlled
Trials Unethical?' (2002) 2:2 Am. J. Bioethics 3 at 5. See also Ezekiel Eman-
uel and Franklin Miller, 'The Ethics of Placebo-Controlled Trials: A Middle
Ground' (2001) 345 New Eng. J. Med. 915.

22 Giesen, 'Civil Liability of Physicians' at 50.

23 Kathleen Cranley Glass and Trudo Lemmens, 'Research Involving
Humans,' in Downie, Caulfield, and Flood, eds., *Canadian Health Law and
Policy*, 459 at 460. See also U.S., National Commission for the Protection of
Human Subjects of Biomedical and Behavioral Research, *The Belmont*

224   Duff R. Waring and Kathleen Cranley Glass

Report: Ethical Principles and Guidelines for the Protection of Human Subjects of Research (Bethesda, MD: Department of Health, Education, and Welfare, 1978) at 3: 'Research and [clinical] practice may be carried on together when research is designed to evaluate the safety and efficacy of therapy. This need not cause any confusion regarding whether or not the activity requires review; the general rule is that if there is any element of research in an activity, that activity should undergo review for the protection of human subjects.'

24 Giesen, 'Civil Liability of Physicians' at 28.
25 Picard and Robertson, *Legal Liability of Doctors and Hospitals* at 195. See *Cryderman v. Ringrose*, (1977) 6 A.R. 21 at 30 (Dist. Ct.), aff'd (1978) 89 D.L.R. (3d) 32 (Alta. C.A.).
26 *Gomez c. Comité exécutif du Conseil des médecins, dentistes et pharmaciens de l'hôpital universitaire de Québec*, [2001] R.J.Q. 2788 (C.A.).
27 Glass and Lemmens, 'Research Involving Humans' at 496.
28 See Giesen, *International Medical Malpractice Law* at ¶ 1134. See also Glass and Lemmens, 'Research Involving Humans' at 479, n.91. In the Canadian case of *Weiss c. Solomon*, [1989] R.J.Q. 731 (Sup. Ct.), the court cited the *Declaration of Helsinki* in assessing the appropriate standard for disclosure in research.
29 BVerfG, BVerfGE 52(1979), 131(170) cited in Geisen, *International Medical Malpractice Law* at 531.
30 Angela Campbell and Kathleen Cranley Glass, 'The Legal Status of Clinical and Ethics Policies, Codes, and Guidelines in Medical Practice and Research' (2001) 46 McGill L.J. 73.
31 782 A.2d 807 (Md. C.A. 2001) [*Grimes*].
32 Ibid. at 835, 814.
33 Ibid. at 849.
34 Ibid. at 849–50.
35 Ibid. at 850, n.39.
36 Ibid. at 850–1, 862.
37 Ibid. at 850.
38 Trudo Lemmens et al., 'CIOMS' Placebo Rule and the Promotion of Negligent Medical Practice' (2004) Eur. J. Health Law 153–74 at 154.
39 *Crits and Crits v. Sylvester.*
40 *Neufeld v. McQuitty* (1979), 18 A.R. 271 at 276 (S.C. (T.D.)).
41 Glass and Waring, 'Effective Trial Design' at 26. See also *Tri-Council Policy Statement*, at 7.4 for six circumstances in which a placebo may be used as a control treatment consistent with clinical equipoise.
42 See Freedman, 'Placebo-Controlled Trials' at 5. Freedman lists 'five broad

classes of cases' in which he thinks placebo controls are both necessary and justified: (1) conditions that have no standard therapy at all; (2) conditions whose standard therapy has been shown to be no better than placebo; (3) conditions whose standard treatment is placebo; (4) conditions whose standard therapy has been called into question by new evidence warranting doubt concerning its presumed net therapeutic advantage; and (5) conditions whose validated optimal treatment is not made freely available to patients, because of cost constraints or otherwise. See also Benjamin Freedman, Charles Weijer, and Kathleen Cranley Glass, 'Placebo Orthodoxy in Clinical Research 1: Empirical and Methodological Myths' (1996) 24 J. L. Med. & Ethics 243 at 247, and Freedman, Glass, and Weijer, 'Placebo Orthodoxy II' at 257 for comments on 'refractory' patient populations which fail to improve on standard treatment.

43 Giesen, *International Medical Malpractice Law* at ¶ 251.
44 Patricia L. Gilbert et al., 'Neuroleptic Withdrawal in Schizophrenic Patients' (1995) 52 Arch. Gen. Psych. 173 at 173, 175, 182–5.
45 Adele C. Viguera et al., 'Clinical Risk Following Abrupt and Gradual Withdrawal of Maintenance Neuroleptic Treatment' (1997) 54 Arch. Gen. Psych. 49 at 49–54.
46 Ross J. Baldessarini et al., 'Medication Removal and Research in Psychotic Disorders' (1998) 55 Arch. Gen. Psych. 281 at 282.
47 Gilbert et al., 'Neuroleptic Withdrawal' at 182.
48 Richard J. Wyatt, 'Neuroleptics and the Natural Course of Schizophrenia' (1991) 17 Schizophrenia Bull. 325; and John F. Greden and Rajiv Tandon, 'Long-Term Treatment for Lifetime Disorders?' (1995) 52 Arch. Gen. Psych. 197 at 198.
49 Greden and Tandon, 'Long-Term Treatment for Lifetime Disorders?'
50 Viguera et al. 'Clinical Risk' at 51.
51 Greden and Tandon, 'Long-Term Treatment for Lifetime Disorders?' Carl Elliott and Charles Weijer, 'Cruel and Unusual Treatment' (1995) 110:10 Saturday Night 31 at 32.
52 Greden and Tandon, 'Long-Term Treatment for Lifetime Disorders?'
53 See Delores King, 'Debatable Forms of Consent,' *Boston Globe*, 16 November 1998, A1. King quotes Wesley Acorn, then president of the national consumer council for the U.S. National Alliance for the Mentally Ill.
54 Baldessarini et al., 'Medication Removal'; Viguera et al., 'Clinical Risk' at 54; Ross J. Baldessarini, 'Risks and Implications of Interrupting Maintenance Psychotropic Drug Therapy' (1995) 63 Psychotherapy and Psychosomatics 137 at 139; Dilip V. Jeste et al., 'Considering Neuroleptic Maintenance and Taper on a Continuum' (1995) 52 Arch. Gen. Psych. 209 at

210; Richard J. Wyatt, 'Risks of Withdrawing Antipsychotic Medications' (1995) 52 Arch. Gen. Psych. 205 at 207.

55 Viguera et al., 'Clinical Risk' at 50.

56 William T. Carpenter and Robert R. Conley, 'Sense and Nonsense: An Essay on Schizophrenia Research Ethics' (1999) 35 Schizophrenia Research 219 at 222.

57 William T. Carpenter, Paul S. Appelbaum, and Robert J. Levine, 'The Declaration of Helsinki and Clinical Trials: A Focus on Placebo-Controlled Trials in Schizophrenia' (2003) 160 Am. J. Psych. 356 at 359.

58 John R. Geddes et al., 'Relapse Prevention with Antidepressant Drug Treatment in Depressive Disorders: A Systematic Review' (2003) 361 Lancet 653.

59 C. Michael Stern and Theodore Pincus, 'Placebo-Controlled Studies in Rheumatoid Arthritis: Ethical Issues' (1999) 353 Lancet 400.

60 Picard and Robertson, *Legal Liability of Doctors and Hospitals* at 218.

61 *Snell v. Farrell*, [1990] 2 S.C.R. 311 at 320, Sopinka J.

62 Picard and Robertson, *Legal Liability of Doctors and Hospitals* at 218, 228.

63 *Snell v. Farrell*, at 313, 327–8.

64 Ibid. at 328–30.

65 Ibid. at 312, 324.

66 *Sentilles v. Inter-Caribbean Shipping Corp.*, 361 U.S. 107 at 109–10 (1959), cited with approval in *Snell v. Farrell* at 331.

67 Picard and Robertson, *Legal Liability of Doctors and Hospitals* at 229.

68 Allen M. Linden, *Canadian Tort Law*, 5th ed. (Markham, ON: Butterworths, 1993) at 363. See also Picard and Robertson, *Legal Liability of Doctors and Hospitals* at 229.

69 Marc A. Rodwin, 'Strains in the Fiduciary Metaphor: Divided Physician Loyalties and Obligations in a Changing Health Care System' (1995) 21 Am. J.L. & Med. 241 at 243.

70 Robertson, 'Negligence and Malpractice' at 106. See also Rodwin, 'Strains in the Fiduciary Metaphor' at 243–7.

71 Robertson, 'Negligence and Malpractice.'

72 Rodwin, 'Strains in the Fiduciary Metaphor' at 247–8.

73 Ibid. at 248.

74 Picard and Robertson, *Legal Liability of Doctors and Hospitals* at 4–6.

75 Mary Marshall and Barbara von Tigerstrom, 'Health Information,' in Downie, Caulfield, and Flood, eds., *Canadian Health Law and Policy* 157 at 188. See *McInerney v. MacDonald*, [1992] 2 S.C.R. 138.

76 Robertson, 'Negligence and Malpractice' at 98. See *Norberg v. Wynrib*, [1992] 2 S.C.R. 226; and *C.D.C. v. Starzecki*, [1996] 2 W.W.R. 317 (Man. Q.B.).

77 *Moore v. The Regents of the University of California,* 793 P.2d 479 at 483, 488, 489 (Cal. 1990).
78 Ibid.
79 Kathleen Cranley Glass and Trudo Lemmens, 'Conflict of Interest and Commercialization of Biomedical Research: What Is the Role of Research Ethics Review?' in Timothy Caulfield and Bryn Williams-Jones, eds., *The Commercialization of Genetic Research: Ethical, Legal and Policy Issues* (New York: Kluwer Academic, 1999), 79.
80 Advisory Committee on Human Radiation Experiments, *The Human Radiation Experiments* (New York: Oxford University Press, 1996).
81 Jerry Menikoff, *Law and Bioethics: An Introduction* (Washington, DC: Georgetown University Press, 2001) at 157, 209.
82 Freedman, Glass, and Weijer, 'Placebo Orthodoxy II' at 254.
83 Temple, 'Problems in Interpreting' at 267–75; Temple and Ellenberg, 'Placebo-Controlled Trials' at 455–63.
84 Arts. 1474, 1477 C.C.Q.
85 Page Keeton et al., eds., *Prosser on the Law of Torts,* 5th ed. (St Paul, MN: West Publishing, 1984) at 484.
86 Ibid. at 482.
87 Menikoff, *Law and Bioethics* at 209.
88 Keeton et al., *Prosser on the Law of Torts* at 490.
89 Paul S. Appelbaum et al., 'False Hopes and Best Data: Consent to Research and the Therapeutic Misconception' (1987) 17 Hastings Center Report 20; Claire Snowdon, Jo Garcia, and Diana Elbourne, 'Making Sense of Randomization: Responses of Parents of Critically Ill Babies to Random Allocation of Treatment in a Clinical Trial' (1997) 45 Soc. Sci. & Med. 1337; Katie Featherstone and Jenny L. Donovan, 'The Struggle to Make Sense of Participating in a Randomized Controlled Trial' (2002) 55 Soc. Sci. & Med. 709.
90 Freedman, Glass, and Weijer, 'Placebo Orthodoxy II' at 254.
91 Glass and Lemmens, 'Research Involving Humans' at 482.
92 *Grimes* at 850.
93 Ibid. at 816, citing Richard W. Garnett, 'Why Informed Consent? Human Experimentation and the Ethics of Autonomy' (1996) 36 Cath. Law. 455 at 458–60.
94 *Norberg* at 315.
95 U.S., President's Commission for the Study of Ethical Problems in Medicine and Biomedical and Behavioral Research, *Compensating Research Subjects* (Washington, DC: Government Printing Office, 1982) at 55–7.

10 Her Majesty's Research Subjects: Liability of the Crown in Research Involving Humans

SANA HALWANI

A number of health crises have recently confronted Canada: the Krever Inquiry into Canada's blood supply,[1] the Walkerton inquiry into water supply in Ontario,[2] and the coroner's investigation into the death of Vanessa Young and the role of the drug regulatory system[3] have all revealed inadequacies in critical regulatory systems. Perhaps partly in response to these crises, the 2002 Speech from the Throne contained a commitment to 'renew federal health protection legislation to better address emerging risks, adapt modern technology and emphasize prevention.'[4] Both the crises and the commitment indicate that there is room to improve the regulatory systems in place to protect our health. In addition, the need to improve the system of protection of human research subjects has also been the subject of intense debate and publication.[5]

While many of these publications have criticized the current governance system of research in Canada and exposed its weaknesses, they generally do not discuss in detail the potential liability of the government resulting from the lack of oversight. In chapter 8 of this volume, Mary Thomson explores the potential liability of researchers, as well as institutions and Research Ethics or Institutional Review Boards (REB/IRBs). In the introduction, she states: 'In the past, research activities have not been the target of liability claims. Lawsuits against researchers have been few. The number and creativity of such claims is increasing, however ...'[6] Recent papers in the *Journal of the American Medical Association* indicate how the research sector in the United States is coming under increasing legal scrutiny[7] and how various legal tools, including those based on tort law, are being employed.[8] In the same spirit, this paper explores the potential liability of the Crown for research activities funded or regulated by the federal government.

Thus far, no claims involving Crown liability for injured research subjects have been brought to the courts. Although mounting a case against the Crown is not as 'simple' as mounting one against researchers, research institutions, or even REB members, there are at least three reasons for considering this option. First, especially if the institutional defendant in an action is a university or a small company, resources may be limited and the defendant may default on a damage award. If the Crown is found to be one of the defendants at fault, it is jointly and severally liable,[9] and the plaintiff will have the benefit of its 'deep pockets.' Second, as Thomson has noted, non-parties cannot be examined prior to trial except with leave, and so a plaintiff's best strategy is to name all possible defendants in the statement of claim.[10] This strategy should allow plaintiffs to examine the federal regulatory or funding body under suspicion. Finally, governance for research involving humans has come under fire as being wholly inadequate to protect research subjects.[11] As McDonald has pointed out, 'At the national level, twice as much is spent on overseeing research involving animals as is spent on research involving humans ... Mice in Canadian laboratories are much better looked after in governance terms than are human subjects.'[12] Arguably, these criticisms have given the Crown notice of the deficiencies of the system; given that the deficiencies are known, inaction would be difficult to excuse.

Since little has been written on this subject, the negligence analysis undertaken here will be based on basic tort and Crown liability principles. First, however, the government agencies that might be considered as defendants, the current state of research regulation in Canada, and the doubts over the adequacy of the current system of oversight will be outlined.

Which Government Agencies?

The two types of federal government agencies that will be discussed in this paper are the federal funding agencies – the Canadian Institutes of Health Research (CIHR), the Natural Sciences and Engineering Research Council (NSERC), and the Social Sciences and Humanities Research Council (SSHRC) – as well as the Therapeutic Products Directorate (TPD), the department responsible for overseeing clinical trial applications. The three funding agencies present similar issues and the CIHR will be used as the model for all three.[13] Other bodies might also be considered, such as provincial funding agencies, or the National

Council on Ethics in Human Research (NCEHR), which is responsible for assisting REBs in a number of capacities, including interpreting and implementing ethics guidelines, and maintaining and developing ethics expertise.[14] The CIHR and TPD have been chosen because they represent the federal government's most important roles in research: funding and regulating.

The Canadian Institutes of Health Research

The CIHR is a Crown corporation that reports to Parliament through the minister of health, via its Governing Council. It was established in 2000 by the *Canadian Institutes of Health Research Act*,[15] as the successor to the Medical Research Council (MRC). Essentially, its objective is to promote health research in Canada,[16] in a similar manner to the National Institutes of Health (NIH) in the United States. In furthering its objective, the CIHR may 'provide funding to promote, assist and undertake health research.'[17] It is primarily this role that is of interest here.

The *CIHR Act* outlines a series of powers and functions for CIHR, including to

(d) monitor, analyze and evaluate issues, including ethical issues, pertaining to health or health research [and]
(e) advise the Minister in respect of any matter relating to health research or health policy.[18]

Under the *CIHR Act*, the Governing Council of the CIHR is required to establish one or more standing committees to advise it, particularly with respect to the purposes outlined above. Thus, a Standing Committee on Ethics (SCE) was established in 2001. The mandate of the SCE includes 'ensuring that research funded by CIHR meets the highest standards of ethics ... [and] ensuring that public accountability and transparency concerns are met, and quality assurance reviews of research ethics operations are carried out.'[19] Since the CIHR's ethical policies in this area are outlined in the *Tri-Council Policy Statement (TCPS)*,[20] one can assume that this is the standard to which the SCE should be holding researchers. In terms of quality assurance of research ethics review, both the *TCPS* and the International Council on Harmonisation, Good Clinical Practice (*ICH-GCP*) guidelines[21] give guidance on the composition and procedures of REBs. In addition, the *TCPS* and *ICH-GCP* guidelines both set substantive conditions to be enforced by REBs in their review of protocols and consent documents.

Although the SCE has a mandate to ensure that research funded by the CIHR is ethical, no committee appears to have the wider mandate of ensuring that CIHR-funded research is safe – or as safe as possible – for research subjects. Ethics review, however, contains an inherent element of 'safety review.' Under the *TCPS* one of the guiding ethical principles is that '[r]esearch subjects must not be subjected to unnecessary risks of harm, and their participation in research must be essential to achieving scientifically and societally important aims that cannot be realized without the participation of human subjects.'[22] Thus, in ensuring that research is ethical, the CIHR should at the same time be ensuring that the risks for research subjects have been minimized.

Apart from the SCE, the CIHR, along with the other federal funding agencies, has established the Interagency Advisory Panel on Research Ethics (PRE).[23] This body has stewardship of the *TCPS*[24] and was created to advise the funding agencies on 'the evolution, interpretation, implementation and educational needs of the TCPS.'[25] The terms of reference of the PRE state that it must report to the presidents of the funding agencies, who in turn decide what action should be taken.[26] The *TCPS* is arguably the most important research ethics policy statement in Canada, and its interpretation and application is critical to the protection of human research subjects. Thus, one could argue that the CIHR's role in the PRE is an inherent part of the CIHR's research ethics mandate.

The PRE is mandated to, inter alia, advise on implementation of the *TCPS* and participate in the dialogue on the development of an oversight system for the ethics review process. Both of these mandates necessarily involve discussion of and investigation into the work of REBs. Thus, the work of the PRE represents the kind of monitoring role the CIHR takes with respect to REBs.

In its 'Proposed Ethics Agenda for CIHR,' the departing MRC Standing Committee on Ethics noted that the CIHR's role in quality assurance of research ethics review is integrally related to the broad function of good corporate practice. It further stated that the disbursement of public funds requires the highest standards of stewardship, which should be fulfilled through a number of means including due diligence of the research proposals to which it grants public funds.[27]

The Therapeutic Products Directorate

The TPD is part of the Health Products and Food Branch (HPFB), which is part of Health Canada, and regulates clinical trials; thus TPD is a government department. Though TPD and CIHR can be characterized differently, both are government entities, and the main differences between them – in terms of legal status – are their relationships to Parliament (one is a government department and the other is a corporation) and their treatment under the *Financial Administration Act*.[28] Neither of these differences is important in the context of this paper, since both are agents of the Crown.[29]

The statutory power of the TPD comes from the *Food and Drug Act*[30] and its Regulations. In 2001, Parliament enacted the *Regulations Amending the Food and Drug Regulations (1024 – Clinical Trials)*[31] to govern the sale and importation of drugs for use in clinical trials. Clinical trials cannot be undertaken lawfully without authorization from the TPD. The regulations outline the conditions that must be met for initial and continuing authorization, including the sponsor's obligations during the trial. The regulations also require the sponsor of a trial to inform the minister of any serious unexpected adverse drug reactions, whether inside or outside of Canada. The TPD has adopted the *ICH-GCP* guidelines, and although these do not have the force of law, they should aid researchers in complying with the 'good clinical practice' requirement in the *Trial Regulations*.

A clinical trial application submitted to the TPD must include an attestation of REB approval, as well as information about the clinical trial site, the investigator, and the drug. A default system is in place such that a trial can commence thirty days after Health Canada has received the application, as long as REB approval has been obtained, even if a 'no objection letter' has not been received.[32] The minister may reject an application if the clinical trial is contrary to the best interests of the clinical trial subjects,[33] or suspend authorization if such action is necessary to prevent injury to the health of a subject, or to another person.[34]

The Health Products and Food Branch Inspectorate is charged with the task of inspecting and enforcing the *Trial Regulations*, thus they may also be a target for tort actions. An inspection strategy has been published by HPFB and states that 'up to 2% of all Canadian clinical trial sites will be inspected each year ... The choice of inspection sites will be reviewed periodically ... and will take into consideration the level of risk to the enrolled subjects, and the observations made during past inspections.'[35] In addition, if a risk of non-compliance is identified, an investigation will be conducted if deemed necessary.[36]

In the Regulatory Impact Analysis Statement of the *Trial Regulations*, Health Canada stated that the framework had been designed, among other things, to 'shorten the time required for clinical trial application review, without endangering the health and safety or Canadians, [and] improve safety mechanisms for clinical trial subjects, such as compliance with generally accepted principles of good clinical practice.'[37] The TPD has thus clearly made the protection of research subjects part of its mandate.

Research Regulation in Canada

As can be seen by the above descriptions, both the TPD and CIHR rely heavily on the REB system of ethics review. A number of problems with REBs and research governance more generally have already been canvassed elsewhere in this volume.[38] Therefore, only two issues relevant to the liability analysis will be flagged in this section.

First, a new development in the world of REBs is the Health Canada REB. Although liability for research reviewed by this REB will not be explored in this paper, establishing liability in this context would likely be easier than when the REB is affiliated with an institution that is not an agent of the Crown. Second, the *TCPS* specifies that research should be subject to review on a continuing basis, at the very least via an annual written report.[39] Ongoing review can take a number of different forms, including review of the consent process, creation of a safety monitoring committee, and review of adverse event reports. Despite the obvious importance of such procedures, few boards seem to be fulfilling this requirement.[40] This kind of omission on the part of an REB should constitute non-compliance with the *TCPS*, thereby causing an institution to lose its funding.

Regardless of the complex web of oversight already in place, some research is not being reviewed at all. Private research that is neither funded by government nor monitored by the drug regulatory process is 'invisible' to the federal government.

Is the Current Oversight System Adequate?

One of the reasons for attempting to establish liability on the part of the Crown is the underlying assumption that the current system of oversight is inadequate. Is this a fair assumption? Evidence of the inadequacy of the current system can be found both directly from Canadian academics and researchers, and indirectly by analogy to the United States.

The Oversight of Research Ethics Boards

McDonald has provided a stinging evaluation of research governance in Canada. Much of his criticism is based on the over-reliance on REBs. He argues that 'The REB process ... has become the reification of the sum total of responsibilities and accountabilities for researchers, research institutions, research sponsors, and research regulators. In effect, this rationalizes the avoidance of major responsibilities that arise before, after and on the peripheries of the REB review process.'[41] Hirtle, Lemmens, and Sprumont have also expressed concern that we may be 'relying too heavily on individual integrity of ethics committee members.'[42] Their reproaches ring true when one considers the critical role played by REBs, as outlined above. This dependence on REBs is more worrying when one notes that REB approval has become focused on consent forms, rather than on a serious review of justice issues and risk/benefit analyses.[43] A reliance on REBs would not pose these problems if accountability and oversight were guaranteed. However, in Canada, very few controls have been placed on the work of ethics committees.

In the United States, the Office for Human Research Protection (OHRP) publishes common findings of non-compliance by researchers, institutions, and members of IRBs, the American equivalent of REBs. These run the gamut from research conducted *without* IRB review, to IRB meetings being convened without quorum, to a failure to obtain legally effective informed consent.[44] The FDA has the power to debar individuals or firms who violate the *Food, Drug and Cosmetics Act*.[45] Debarment, which may be permanent or for a designated time, results in individuals no longer being able to participate in drug trials.[46]

At least one Canadian university has been found non-compliant with the requirements of the U.S. federal regulations on a number of counts, including inadequate informed consent documents and continuing review.[47] However, even in the United States, regulatory oversight has been characterized as inadequate because of a focus on paperwork rather than the actual operation of the IRBs.[48]

The System of Review

REB members themselves have misgivings about the system of review. In Beagan's interviews with such members, approximately half of them were significantly concerned about the effectiveness of review.[49] For example, one member noted that as compared with the highly regulated use of animals in research, 'We don't have a clue how many humans were enrolled [in research in Canada last year].'[50] In addition, one REB member had been involved in a study on previous research subjects' perceptions of the consent process. The study showed that patients simply acquiesced to their doctors and did not actually understand the process.[51]

In the McCusker et al. study of the clinical research monitoring system implemented at St Mary's Hospital Centre in Montreal, many problems were revealed by the ethics committee. For example, when consent form audits were performed, 22 per cent of hospital charts of patients in hospital research were missing consent forms.[52] When interviews were conducted with research subjects, 19 per cent had little understanding of experimental treatments and procedures, or of the risks and benefits associated with the research in which they were involved.[53] These findings indicate that hospitals may not be complying with some of the minimum requirements for ethical research.

There are also clear problems with adverse events reporting. In the United States, Adil Shamoo has argued that the majority of adverse events are not reported.[54] There is no reason to believe that the situation is any different in Canada. This lack of reporting is critical because it prevents information about what can and does go wrong during research to be available to those who might be able to prevent future adverse events.

Taken together, these findings do not demonstrate egregious violations of guidelines and regulations, but they do give cause for concern. One should remember that researchers need not be acting in bad faith to harm patients.

The Status of Research Ethics Boards

Although the status of REBs in Canadian law cannot be fully explored in this paper, I will briefly highlight the importance of this issue. As REBs are now mentioned in statutes, such as the Alberta *Health Information Act*,[55] and regulations, such as the *Trial Regulations*, one can reasonably ask whether they can be characterized as government bodies subject to administrative law. In the clinical trial context – where trials can proceed after a thirty-day default period has elapsed as long as REB approval has been obtained – the responsibility for ensuring safety is in effect, at least in part, delegated to REBs. Thus, the regulations 'provide Federal recognition of the important service provided by REBs.'[56]

Although review boards are being given increasing recognition and responsibility by governments, there is still no accreditation system for REBs in Canada. This state of affairs is under review, and as the *Trial Regulations'* Regulatory Impact Analysis Statement explains: 'The policy evaluation conducted clearly identified the need to have a formal accreditation system for REBs. An accreditation system would promote compliance with good clinical practice.' The evident lack of governance in this area not only creates concerns for the safety of research subjects but may also play a role in the Crown liability analysis, as will be discussed below.

Crown Liability for Harm to Research Subjects

A large number of scenarios of potential Crown liability might be explored in this paper. To narrow them down, a number of 'impossible' scenarios will first be eliminated. First, research without a Crown connection, that, is unregulated private research, cannot draw Crown liability. In such a case, the Crown has made a decision not to regulate or oversee research in a specific sector, and the courts cannot oblige it to do so.[57]

Second, in most circumstances, a research subject will only be able to argue liability on the part of the Crown if there has *also* been wrongdoing on the part of the researcher or REB members. This assumption follows from the fact that the Crown generally has an oversight function and can only be found liable for not preventing or stopping the negligent conduct of the other players involved in research. For example, if there has been no REB approval of the research and a research subject is harmed because of a serious flaw in the protocol, the researcher will be at fault, and the Crown may also be at fault for not having verified that REB approval was obtained.

Third, as most research presents inherent risks, it is inevitable that some subjects may be injured, even if all the parties involved in research act in a non-negligent manner. Thus, just as a doctor will not be found negligent if he or she has lived up to the standards of her profession, so the Crown cannot be held liable if it has exercised a sufficient amount of oversight. What 'sufficient' might mean in this context will be explored in detail below.

Thus the generic scenario is as follows: a research subject is harmed in CIHR-funded research or in a clinical drug trial approved by the TPD; the harm is caused at least in part by a failure of the researcher and/or the REB; and this failure is against TPD regulation or the *TCPS*. Issues particular to either the CIHR or TPD will be explored after a general discussion of Crown liability, and more specifics will be discussed when necessary to refine the analysis.

Crown Liability: Generally

Originally, at common law the Crown could not be sued. This situation has changed gradually over the years and today, the *Crown Liability and Proceedings Act (CLPA)* imposes tort liability on the federal Crown.[58] Although this statute enables parties to sue the Crown, it also places a number of limits on potential liability.

Liability in tort is imposed by section 3 of the *CLPA*:

> 3. The Crown is liable for the damages for which, if it were a person, it would be liable
> > (b) in any other province [other than Quebec] in respect of
> > > (i) a tort committed by a servant of the Crown, or
> > > (ii) a breach of duty attaching to the ownership, occupation, possession or control of property.

In the context of research, only section 3(a) will apply, as Crown property will not be involved.

The Crown is like a corporation; it can only act through human servants. As Hogg explains, 'this does not usually cause difficulty in the creation of rights and duties because the doctrines of agency and vicarious liability can be used by or against the Crown to hold it bound by the acts of its servants or agents.'[59] In addition, under section 2 of the *CLPA*, 'servant' is defined as including agent. Vicarious liability for the Crown's agents and servants can therefore be imposed if they are acting in the course of employment, and if there would be a cause of action in tort against them personally.[60] Thus, establishing Crown liability requires (1) establishing liability on the part of a Crown servant and (2) linking the actions of the servant to the Crown.

NEGLIGENCE OF THE SERVANT

As with all negligence actions, establishing liability for a servant requires the finding of a duty, the breaching of the relevant standard of care, and causation between the breach and the harm. A two-step test has been adopted in *Kamloops* to establish a duty of care. The court must ask: '(1) is there a sufficiently close relationship between the parties (the [defendant] and the person who has suffered the damage) so that, in the reasonable contemplation of the [defendant], carelessness on its part might cause damage to that person? If so (2) are there considerations which ought to negative or limit (a) the scope of the duty and (b) the class of persons to whom it is owed or (c) the damages to which a breach of it may give rise?[61] Although any claim that would arise in the scenario imagined here will be novel, the 'categories of negligence are never closed.'[62] If foreseeability and proximity are established, then a duty of care is owed unless there are considerations to limit it. Establishing a breach of the standard of care and demonstrating causation are fact-specific and so their analysis will be taken up again below for the specific cases of TPD and CIHR employees.

THE LINK TO THE CROWN

An important first step in linking any negligent action to the Crown is to establish that the act was committed by a Crown servant. The Crown includes government departments headed by a minister, the minister providing the necessary link. Entities that perform governmental functions are not agents of the Crown unless a statute designates them as such.[63] Thus the reason why the Crown cannot be held vicariously liable for the negligence of REB members is because neither hospitals nor universities (the usual institutions that house REBs) are controlled by a minister or declared agents of the Crown. The TPD, however, is controlled by the minister of health and the CIHR is declared a Crown agent by its statute.[64]

In general, the case law assimilates a Crown agent into an individual Crown servant. Thus the Crown, not the agent, is vicariously liable for the actions of the agent's employees. The agent is not itself a master.[65] Because of this rule, employees of the TPD and CIHR are in the same position relative to the Crown: both can create vicarious liability for the Crown.

Immunity clauses may relieve Crown servants or the Crown from liability; however, no immunities have been enacted for TPD employees in the *Food and Drug Act* or its Regulations, or for CIHR employees in the *CIHR Act*. Therefore, the Crown should be liable if the tortious actions of their employees cause damages.

Recently, research subjects in a melanoma cancer study in the United States brought a claim against investigators, members of IRBs, and institutions involved in the research. In granting the defendant's motion to dismiss, the U.S. District Court for the Northern District of Oklahoma held that there is no private right of action under the *Federal Policy for the Protection of Human Subjects*[66] because a comprehensive enforcement scheme is provided by the Food and Drug Administration (FDA).[67] This approach has not been adopted in Canada: the possibility of finding the Crown liable therefore remains.

For vicarious liability to arise, the tort must be committed 'in the course of employment.' Although this does not mean that the Crown must have specifically authorized the act, the act must be 'closely connected with the duties of employment.'[68] Over the years, the courts have grappled with this concept. For example, the Crown has been held liable for a supervisor's intentional infliction of nervous shock on a subordinate, because the actions of the supervisor were directly related to his duties.[69] However, the Crown cannot be held liable for the unlawful acts of its employees.[70] In the scenario presented here, the actions or omissions of CIHR or TPD employees should be considered 'closely connected' to their duties if, for example, they negligently review a funding or clinical trial application.

Interestingly, although a plaintiff must show that a private duty of care is owed by a Crown servant to establish liability, the *individual* servant does not need to be sued, and identifying the actual tortfeasor is not essential.[71] Thus, the Crown is liable for the collective act or omission of a number of individual Crown servants, for example, the decision of a committee.[72] This may become important if a committee makes funding decisions or a group of inspectors enforce drug trial regulations.

Section 10 of the *CLPA* acts to limit the scope of liability of the Crown by precluding corporate liability on the part of the Crown, and focusing on a private duty of care owed by a servant of the Crown. An act can be insulated from liability if it is characterized as a policy decision and therefore a legitimate exercise of the Crown's discretionary power. Once a prima facie duty of care is established, this policy/operational distinction provides an important way of limiting liability.

The main reason for such a distinction is that the courts are not competent to evaluate the planning decisions of an elected body. As Hogg has explained: 'Obviously, planning decisions differ only in degree from the operational decisions, but operational decisions are those that are more specific, and therefore susceptible to judicial evaluation by reference to the negligence standard of reasonable care.'[73] Thus, when the HPFB inspectorate designs a policy whereby only 2 per cent of trials are to be inspected,[74] that decision cannot be found to be tortious even if it results in injury as long as it has been made on legitimate policy grounds such as the rationing of scarce resources. In *Kamloops*, Wilson J. explained the concept of a 'legitimate' decision in this manner: 'inaction for no reason or inaction for an improper reason cannot be a policy decision taken in the *bona fide* exercise of discretion. Where the question whether the requisite action should be taken has not even been considered by the public authority, or at least has not been considered in good faith, it seems clear that for that very reason the authority has not acted with reasonable care.'[75] Thus, if a government servant's failure to act is not the product of a considered decision, liability will be ascribed if the other elements of negligence are present.

Once a policy is established, a litigant may attack the system as not having been adopted in a bona fide exercise of discretion and demonstrate that under the circumstances, including budgetary restraints, it is appropriate for a court to make a finding on the issue. In *Just v. British Columbia*, a case concerning a system of highway inspection set up by the province, the court stated that a bona fide exercise of discretion requires the authorities to 'specifically consider whether to inspect and if so, the system of inspection must be a reasonable one in all the circumstances.'[76]

Crown Liability: CIHR

In a discussion of the liability of the Medical Research Council (MRC, the predecessor to the CIHR), Sava et al. stated that 'insofar as the MRC assesses information regarding the protocol on the grant application and conducts an ethical review, it is imposed with a similar duty as the institution or the REB ... [It] therefore owes a duty of care to research subjects with respect to its protocol review functions.'[77] In addition to protocol review, the CIHR, like the MRC, is a sponsor of research and this additional function may also establish a duty of care.

Establishing a duty on the part of SCE members requires a finding of foreseeability of harm and of proximity to the research subject.[78] It should be readily foreseeable that funding a research project without

ensuring that it is ethical or that ethics review is being properly conducted could lead to the harm of research subjects. This conclusion is
further supported by the fact that effective ethics review includes a
review of the risks involved.

Proximity has been defined as including two components: reasonable foreseeability of reliance by the defendant and reasonable reliance
by the plaintiff.[79] In *Just*,[80] a highway leading to a popular ski resort
was found to constitute an invitation to use the highway, which gave
rise to a duty of care. In a similar manner, by funding a research
project, the CIHR invites the public to participate in it. It is then reasonable for research subjects to rely on the SCE to ensure the safety of the
research. Essentially, the CIHR is in the position of a research sponsor
and this relationship should provide the required degree of proximity
to research subjects. The invitation is all the more present if the CIHR is
mentioned as a sponsor of the research on the consent form.

The standard to which members of the SCE should be held to might
arise from the *TCPS*. If protocol reviews are being conducted by members of the SCE (or other CIHR employees), then they must be done in
a non-negligent manner and the *TCPS* will be evidence of the relevant
standard of care. In addition, since the CIHR expects funded institutions to comply with the *TCPS*, it might be required to verify that the
institutions are in fact doing so. Although it is unlikely that a court
would find that the SCE should oversee the research projects themselves, it might find that it should monitor the work of REBs. The mandate of the SCE could also provide evidence of this standard of care.

As outlined above, the CIHR has the power to monitor ethical
issues.[81] To that end, it has established the SCE and has given it the
mandate to ensure that research funded by the CIHR meets the highest
standards of ethics and that quality assurance reviews of REBs are carried out.[82] The SCE mandate is outlined in a CIHR by-law. Although a
standing committee oversees the CIHR funding itself, it has not been
mandated to perform ethics review. Thus, the decisions of the SCE are
those most prone to be reviewed in the event of injury to a research
subject. Since the litigant must establish vicarious, not direct, liability,
statutory duties will only be considered as *evidence* of the existence of a
common law duty, not as proof.[83] Thus the breach of a statute or regulation per se does not give rise to liability.

Although statutory power does not create an affirmative duty to act,
it does contain an element of duty.[84] Since a collective act can give rise
to Crown liability, the fact that a negligent decision was made by a

committee should not be a bar unless that decision is characterized as a policy decision.

In addition to statutory duties, a court might look to policies and guidelines promulgated by the CIHR or SCE, such as the *Standing Committee on Ethics – Terms of Reference* and the *TCPS*, in determining the applicable standard of care. It may also look to the reports generated by the PRE on the interpretation and implementation of the *TCPS*. The status of these kinds of soft law instruments has become the subject of academic debate and judicial scrutiny.

As Sossin and Smith have written, 'Soft law cannot in theory bind decision-makers, yet in practice it often has as much or more influence than legislative standards.'[85] Although their work focused on the importance of soft law in the judicial review context, they also commented on the legal status of soft law more generally:

> Soft law, while it may be treated as binding internally, cannot give rise to externally enforceable rights. Canadian jurisprudence recognizes that regulators may, without any specific statutory authority, issue guidelines and other non-binding instruments. Decision-making bodies and ministries must be cautious not to fetter their own discretion by adopting fixed rules of policy in the absence of specific statutory rule-making authority. Nor should guidelines be treated as rules to be applied in every case.[86]

Glass and Campbell have also discussed the legal status of soft law, focusing on the medical practice and research contexts. Echoing the view of Sossin and Smith, they stated, 'while in theory courts are not bound to follow professional standards and norms, they are unlikely to disregard them when they are supported and endorsed within the professional community.'[87] Therefore, although litigants cannot argue that any relevant policies were binding on the CIHR and SCE, they can argue that these policies should inform the court's interpretation of the standard of care by which to evaluate CIHR and SCE action or inaction.

Memoranda of Understanding: Passing the Buck?

One factor that might complicate this part of the analysis is that the CIHR requires institutions receiving funding to sign 'Memoranda of Understanding' attesting that they will, at a minimum, follow the *TCPS*.[88] The CIHR may then argue that by adopting such a requirement it has made a policy decision that cannot be scrutinized by the courts; that is, the CIHR may argue that it has made a policy decision to defer review responsibilities to institutions, and this policy decision insulates it from liability. However, it is difficult to characterize these memoranda as enabling the CIHR to 'monitor ... ethical issues.'[89] Thus, a litigant may challenge the fact that the decision is a bona fide exercise of discretion.

In addition, the memorandum reiterates that the CIHR has 'a responsibility and an obligation to establish and manage policies and programs that enable [it] to fulfil [its] mandate as defined by [the *CIHR Act*],' and the CIHR must 'review the relevant policies of Institutions that wish to be declared eligible to receive [CIHR] funding to ensure that these policies meet TCPS requirements.'[90] Therefore, the memorandum does not appear to create new legal rights for research subjects, nor does it negate any of their already existing rights. First, the memorandum of understanding is a contract between grant or award holders and the CIHR. This means that the CIHR cannot be sued by research subjects on the basis of this document, as they are not parties to the contract. Second, the CIHR's responsibilities – as they have been outlined above – are not delegated to the award holders in the memorandum, but rather, are expressly stated as remaining part of the CIHR's mandate. Thus, overall, the memorandum should be viewed as affecting the position of the CIHR with respect to award holders but not with respect to research subjects.

Generally, even if SCE members, or CIHR employees more generally, are not ensuring that each research project funded is ethical or are not overseeing the operation of REBs in the institutions funded, they will not be held liable if these omissions are part of a well-founded policy, based, for example, on the lack of resources. It is important to realize that persons at all levels of authority can make policy decisions.[91] The nature of the decision is the deciding factor; thus decisions made by the SCE (as opposed to the minister of health or the Governing Council of CIHR) may be characterized as policy decisions by the courts.

If, however, a decision is made to establish a system of protocol review, or a system of REB spot-checks, then they must not be negligently performed. For example, under such circumstances, SCE members could not simply approve problematic protocols or turn a blind eye to an REB that was not conducting continuing review. If harm were caused by these omissions, then the final requirement of causation would be fulfilled, and negligence would be shown.[92]

Crown Liability: TPD

Establishing a duty of care on the part of TPD employees or HPFB inspectors should be simpler than for CIHR employees or SCE members. Since the analysis is similar, only relevant differences will be discussed below.

The TPD is the gatekeeper for clinical trials; trials cannot be initiated without its authorization. Therefore, if that authorization is given negligently, the courts should impose liability. In *Swinamer v. Nova Scotia (Attorney General)*, the Supreme Court held that once the province had built highways, a prima facie duty was created to maintain those highways with due care.[93] Thus, once an approval process has been created, the TPD must administer it with due care. The foreseeability and proximity requirements are fulfilled in a similar manner as stated above for the the CIHR. Approval is an invitation to research subjects to participate, and if an unsafe trial is approved, harm is foreseeable.

Establishing a standard of care might be done by analogy to other inspection or licensing systems established by government. In *Swanson v. Canada (Minister of Transport)*, negligence arose from the acceptance by air safety inspectors of the airline's promise to comply with the specifications in its operating licence; reliance on promises of compliance was inconsistent with the function of ensuring air passenger safety.[94] One of the requirements of the clinical trial application is that REB approval be obtained and that the trial be conducted in accordance with *ICH-GCP* guidelines. A litigant could argue that relying on an assurance by the trial sponsor that both of these conditions have been met is inconsistent with the goal of ensuring safety for clinical trial subjects.

As has been discussed above, REBs bear most of the burden of ensuring that clinical trials are safe and ethical. One might argue that because the Crown relies on REBs to ensure that the rights of subjects are respected, and their safety is duly protected, the Crown would have to adopt a system of REB accreditation or governance more generally to meet its standard of care.

Even if a duty and a breach of standard were established, a litigant would still have to convince the court that the act or omission in question was not part of TPD policy. The TPD has established policies at different stages of the regulatory process, during application review and during the clinical trial itself. Two of these will create hurdles for potential litigants: the thirty-day default system and the inspection policy. Both policies limit the scope of potential TPD liability and the only way that they can be challenged is by demonstrating that they are not a reasonable exercise of discretion.

The thirty-day default system means that if a clinical trial subject is harmed in a trial that has not been reviewed by TPD because it was automatically approved after thirty days, the subject would not be able to argue that this omission was negligent because it was within the scope of the *Trial Regulations*. The subject could try to argue that this policy is unreasonable, but courts have tended not to be open to such arguments, especially when the policy has underlying economic and political reasons.

In a similar manner, since the HPFB inspectorate has stated that a maximum of 2 per cent of trials will be inspected, if a subject was harmed in a trial that was not inspected, the Crown would be immune. It would be even more difficult to argue that this is an unreasonable policy because it is in line with FDA policy in the United States.[95]

Finally, the TPD's (or Health Canada's) decision not to create a system of REB accreditation might also be considered a policy decision by the courts. A counter-argument to that position would be that the policy decision made by the TPD was the decision to include REB approval as part of the clinical trial application process, and that the lack of governance is in fact an operational default that creates liability for the Crown. This argument is bolstered by the fact that the federal government has recognized that some REBs 'do not have the expertise or funding to ensure that drug trials can be conducted according to generally accepted principles of good clinical practice.'[96] Although the government also stated that those REBs should concentrate their efforts in other fields, there remains a very real chance that unqualified REBs will continue to review clinical trial applications and potentially expose research subjects to unreasonable risks. This chance would be reduced if a system of REB governance were put in place.

All in all, the most likely situation that would result in liability is one in which a clinical trial application was reviewed by a TPD employee who negligently authorized it, or if a TPD employee was tipped off that a particular clinical trial was putting subjects at risk and did nothing to follow up. Obviously, causation would have to be shown in the context of the particular trial and injury.

Conclusion

The foregoing analysis does not draw a clear path to Crown liability for an injured research subject. There are numerous difficulties in mounting a case against the Crown for injury resulting from research that it has funded or authorized. The major hurdles appear to be the establishing of a novel duty – from research reviewer to research subject – and the characterization of the negligent action or omission as operative and not policy in nature. The issue of causation, which could not be dealt with fully in the abstract, may also provide substantial obstacles.

Between the two government bodies discussed here, employees within the drug regulatory system appear to be easier targets, primarily because other types of regulatory systems have come under fire and analogies can be drawn to these cases. Apart from the difficulties associated with the novel nature of a claim against the CIHR, courts may be less likely to extend liability to a funding agency if they perceive that such decisions will discourage government from sponsoring research.

Some critics oppose the extension of Crown liability by arguing that the government should not be excessively hindered by the courts. However, negligence should not be insulated from legal liability by the policy-making role of public authorities. Although court action – or the threat of it – can only push reform so far, it will hopefully go some distance to ensuring greater institutional responsibility towards research subjects, as well as greater transparency and accountability.

NOTES

The author thanks Trudo Lemmens and Paul B. Miller for reading and commenting on an earlier draft of this paper.

1 Commission of Inquiry on the Blood System in Canada (Krever Commission), *Final Report* (Ottawa: Public Works and Government Services Canada, 1997), http://www.hc-sc.gc.ca/english/protection/krever/index.html. The commission investigated the contamination of Canada's national blood supply with HIV and Hepatitis C in the late 1970s and 1980s.
2 Walkerton Commission of Inquiry, *Report of the Walkerton Inquiry*, Parts 1 and 2 (Toronto: Queen's Printer for Ontario, 2003), http://www.attorney-general.jus.gov.on.ca/english/about/pubs/walk erton/. The commission investigated the contamination of Walkerton's water supply with *E. coli* bacteria in May 2000, during which 7 people died and 2,300 became ill.
3 Health Products and Food Branch, Health Canada, *Response to the Recom-*

mendations to Health Canada of the Coroner's Jury Investigation into the Death of Vanessa Young (Ottawa: Health Canada, 2002), http://www.hc-sc.gc.ca/ english/protection/vanessa_young/index.html. The coroner's jury investigated the death of a teenager, Vanessa Young, who died after taking the stomach drug Prepulsid; the drug was taken off the market after her death. The investigation indicated that Canada's drug surveillance system may not be effective at detecting adverse drug reactions once the drug is marketed.

4 Canada, Privy Council Office, *The Canada We Want,* Speech from the Throne to Open the Second Session of the Thirty-Seventh Parliament of Canada, 30 September 2002, http://www.pco-bcp.gc.ca/default.asp?Language=E &Page=InformationResources&sub=sf tddt&doc=sftddt2002_e.htm.

5 See, e.g., Simon Verdun-Jones and David N. Weisstub, 'The Regulation of Biomedical Research Experimentation in Canada: Developing an Effective Apparatus for the Implementation of Ethical Principles in a Scientific Milieu' (1996–7) 28 Ottawa L. Rev. 297; Michael McDonald, ed., *The Governance of Health Research Involving Human Subjects* (Ottawa: Law Commission of Canada, 2000); Kathleen Cranley Glass and Trudo Lemmens, 'Research Involving Humans,' in Timothy Caulfield, Jocelyn Downie, and Colleen Flood, eds., *Canadian Health Law and Policy,* 2nd ed. (Markham, ON: Butterworths, 2002); Charles Weijer, 'Placebo Trials and Tribulations' (2002) 166 Can. Med. Assoc. J. 603.

6 Mary M. Thomson, 'Bringing Research into Therapy: Liability Anyone?' in this volume, at 183.

7 Paul E. Kalb and Kristin Graham Koehler, 'Legal Issues in Scientific Research' (2002) 287 J. Am. Med. Assoc. 85.

8 David M. Studdert, Michelle M. Mello, and Troyen A. Brennan, 'Medical Monitoring for Pharmaceutical Injuries: Tort Law for the Public's Health?' (2003) 289 J. Am. Med. Assoc. 889.

9 *Negligence Act,* R.S.O. 1990, c. N.1, s. 1. The federal *Crown Liability and Proceedings Act* imposing liability in tort on the federal Crown has been interpreted as incorporating by reference the law of torts of the province in which the cause of action arose (Peter W. Hogg, *Liability of the Crown,* 2nd ed. [Toronto: Carswell, 1989] at 228). When necessary, I will generally refer to Ontario law in this paper.

10 Thomson, 'Bringing Research into Therapy' at 183–4.

11 See McDonald, *Governance of Health Research Involving Human Subjects.*

12 Michael McDonald, 'Canadian Governance of Health Research Involving Human Subjects: Is Anybody Minding the Store?' (2001) 9 Health L.J. 1 at ¶ 29.

13 The CIHR is being used as the model because it is the agency most likely to fund research that involves health risks to human subjects.

14 NCEHR's full *Terms of Reference* can be found at http://www.ncehr .medical.org/english/mstr_frm.html.

15 R.S.C. 2000, c. 6 [*CIHR Act*].

16 Ibid., s. 4.

17 Ibid., s. 26(a).

18 Ibid., s. 5.

19 Canadian Institutes of Health Research, *Standing Committee on Ethics, Terms of Reference*, http://www.cihr-irsc.gc.ca/e/about/6995.shtml [*SCE Terms*].

20 Medical Research Council, Natural Sciences and Engineering Research Council, and Social Sciences and Humanities Research Council, *Tri-Council Policy Statement: Ethical Conduct for Research Involving Humans* (Ottawa: Public Works and Government Services Canada, 1998), http:// www.pre.ethics.gc.ca/english/policystatement/policystatem ent.cfm [*TCPS*]. The *TCPS* is the closest thing to a national policy on research involving humans that Canada has. The three councils are the Medical Research Council (now superseded by the CIHR), the Natural Sciences and Engineering Research Council, and the Social Sciences and Humanities Research Council. The policy only applies to institutions receiving funding from one of these three granting councils. It has hardly been revised since August 1998.

21 Health Canada, Therapeutic Products Directorate, *Good Clinical Practice: Consolidated Guideline* (Ottawa: Public Works and Government Services Canada, 1997) [*ICH-GCP*].

22 *TCPS* 21 at i.5.

23 It has been suggested that clinical practice guideline developers might be held liable if reliance on those guidelines resulted in harm to a patient (Janet E. Pelly et al., 'Clinical Practice Guidelines Before the Law: Sword or Shield?' 169 Med. J. Austl. 348 at 349). Although the *TCPS* does not establish clinical practice, an analogy could be made to ethics review 'practice.'

24 *TCPS*.

25 See http://www.pre.ethics.gc.ca/english/aboutus/aboutus.cfm.

26 Interagency Advisory Panel on Research, *Terms of Reference: Governance Structure for the Tri-Council Policy Statement*, http://www.pre.ethics.gc.ca/ english/aboutus/termsofreference.cfm.

27 Medical Research Council, Standing Committee on Ethics, *A Proposed Ethics Agenda for CIHR: Challenges and Opportunities* (March 2000), http:// www.cihr-irsc.gc.ca/e/about/ethics_mrc_standing_committee_e.pdf at 6.

28 R.S.C. 1985, c. F-10.

29 The agency of the TPD and CIHR is explained above at 231.

30 R.S.C. 2001 (4th Supp.), c. 42

31 S.O.R./2001-203 [*Trial Regulations*].

32 Ibid., s. C.05.006.

33 Ibid., s. C.05.006(b)(ii)(B).

34 Ibid., s. C.05.017(1).

35 Health Products and Food Branch Inspectorate, *Inspection Strategy for Clinical Trials* (Ottawa: Health Canada, 2002), http://www.hc-sc.gc.ca/hpfb-dgpsa/inspectorate/insp_strat_clin_tria_tc_e.html at 6 [*Inspection Strategy*].

36 Ibid. at 8.

37 Regulations Amending the Food and Drug Regulations (1024–Clinical Trials) Regulatory Impact Analysis Statement, C. Gaz. 2001.II.1129, http://www.hc-sc.gc.ca/hpfb-dgpsa/inspectorate/food_drug_reg_amend_1024_gcp_e.pdf [*Regulatory Impact Analysis Statement*].

38 See Kathleen Cranley Glass, 'Questions and Challenges in the Governance of Research Involving Humans: A Canadian Perspective,' in this volume, at 43.

39 *Good Clinical Practice: Consolidated Guideline*, Art. 1.13.

40 Charles Weijer, 'Continuing Review of Research Approved by Canadian Research Ethics Boards' (2001) 164 Can. Med. Assoc. J. 1305 at 1305.

41 'Canadian Governance of Health Research Involving Human Subjects' at ¶ 20.

42 Marie Hirtle, Trudo Lemmens, and Dominique Sprumont, 'A Comparative Analysis of Research Ethics Review Mechanisms and the ICH Good Clinical Practice Guideline' (2000) 7 Eur. J. Health L. 265 at 273.

43 Brenda Beagan, 'Ethics Review for Human Subjects Research: Interviews with Members of Research Ethics Boards and National Organizations,' in McDonald, ed., *Governance of Health Research Involving Humans* at 188. See also Charles Weijer, 'The Ethical Analysis of Risk' (2000) 28 J.L. Med. and Ethics 244.

44 OHRP, Compliance Oversight Branch, Division of Human Subject Protections, *OHRP Compliance Activities: Common Findings and Guidance: 7/10/2002*, http://ohrp.osophs.dhhs.gov/references/findings.pdf.

45 21 U.S.C. §335(a) and (b) (1997).

46 The debarment list is published by Office of Regulatory Affairs of the FDA, <http://www.fda.gov/ora/compliance_ref/debar/default.htm>.

47 Letter from OHRP to Raelene Rathbone, McMaster University (22 January 2001), http://ohrp.osophs.dhhs.gov/detrm_letrs/jan01f.pdf. Canadian institutions are required to comply with U.S. regulations when they receive U.S. funding.

48 Hirtle, Lemmens, and Sprumont, 'Comparative Analysis' at 274–5. See also damning reports of the Department of Health and Human Services' Office of Inspector General: Office of Inspector General, *Institutional Review Boards: Their Role in Reviewing Approved Research* (Washington, DC: Department of Health and Human Services, 1998); Office of Inspector General, *Institutional Review Boards: Promising Approaches* (Washington, DC: Department of Health and Human Services, 1998); Office of Inspector General, *Institutional Review Boards: The Emergence of Independent Boards* (Washington, DC: Department of Health and Human Services, 1998); and Office of Inspector General, *Institutional Review Boards: A Time for Reform* (Washington, DC: Department of Health and Human Services, 1998).

49 Beagan, 'Ethics Review' at 186.

50 Ibid. at 187.

51 Ibid. at 188.

52 Jane McCusker et al., 'Monitoring Clinical Research: Report of One Hospital's Experience' (2001) 164 Can. Med. Assoc. J. 1321 at 1323.

53 Ibid. at 1324.

54 Adil E. Shamoo, 'Adverse Events Reporting: The Tip of an Iceberg' (2001) 8 Accountability in Research 197.

55 R.S.A. 2000, c. H-5.

56 *Regulatory Impact Analysis Statement* at 1142. See Trudo Lemmens and Benjamin Freedman, 'Ethics Review for Sale? Conflict of Interest and Commercial Research Review Boards' (2000) 78 Milbank Quarterly 547; Trudo Lemmens and Alison Thompson, 'Noninstitutional Commercial Review Boards in North America: A Critical Appraisal and Comparison with IRBs' (2001) 23 IRB 1.

57 This relates to the operational/policy distinction that will be explored further below.

58 R.S.C. 1985, c. C-50 [*CLPA*]. Only the federal Crown is relevant, as the Crown agencies under scrutiny are federal. If provincial agencies were at issue, provincial Crown liability statutes would be pertinent.

59 Hogg, *Liability of the Crown* at 12.

60 David Sgayias et al., *The Annotated 1995 Crown Liability and Proceedings Act* (Toronto: Carswell, 1994) at 16. The necessity for a private duty of care owed by a particular servant or agent arises from s. 10 of the *CLPA*.

61 *City of Kamloops v. Nielsen*, [1984] 2 S.C.R. 2 at 10–11 [*Kamloops*].

62 *Donoghue v. Stevenson*, [1932] AC 562 (H.L.) at 619.

63 Hogg, *Liability of the Crown* at 10.

64 *CIHR Act*, s. 3(2).

65 Hogg, *Liability of the Crown* at 257.

66 45 C.F.R. 46 (2001).

67 *Robertson v. McGee*, 2002 U.S. Dist. LEXIS 4072 (N.D. Okla., 2002). The court cited a US. Supreme Court case (*Merrell Dow Pharmaceuticals v. Thompson*, 478 U.S. 804 (1986)) in support of this principle.

68 Ibid. at 93.

69 *Boothman v. Canada*, [1993] 3 F.C. 381 (T.D.).

70 *Levesque v. Rockefeller*, [1991] 1 F.C. D-2 (T.D.).

71 Hogg, *Liability of the Crown* at 88.

72 *Wilfrid Nadeau Inc. v. The Queen*, [1977] 1 F.C. 541 (T.D.), aff'd [1980] 1 F.C. 808 (C.A.).

73 Hogg, *Liability of the Crown* at 129.

74 *Inspection Strategy.*

75 *Kamloops* at 24.

76 *Just v. British Columbia*, [1989] 2 S.C.R. 1228 at ¶ 21.

77 Helen Sava, P. Theodore Matlow, and Michael J. Sole, 'Legal Liability of Physicians in Medical Research' (1994) 17:2 Clin. and Invest. Med. 148 at 174.

78 The traditional tort law foreseeability test (*Donoghue v. Stevenson*) has been refined by the Supreme Court of Canada in *Canadian National Railway v. Norsk Pacific Steamship*, [1992] 1 S.C.R. 1021 to incorporate 'proximity' as an additional criterion to establish a prima facie duty of care in the first step of the *Kamloops* test.

79 *Hercules Management Ltd. v. Ernst and Young*, [1997] 2 S.C.R. 165 [*Hercules*].

80 *Just v. British Columbia.*

81 *CIHR Act*, s. 5(d),

82 *SCE Terms.*

83 *R. v. Saskatchewan Wheat Pool*, [1983] 1 S.C.R. 205.

84 Hogg, *Liability of the Crown* at 130.

85 Lorne Sossin and Charles W. Smith, 'Hard Choices and Soft Law: Ethical Codes, Policy Guidelines and the Role of the Courts in Regulating Government' (2003) 40 Alta. L. Rev. 867 at 869.

86 Ibid. at 888.

87 Angela Campbell and Kathleen Cranley Glass, 'The Legal Status of Clinical and Ethics Policies, Codes and Guidelines in Medical Practice and Research' (2001) 46 McGill L.J. 473.

88 Canadian Institutes of Health Research, Natural Sciences and Engineering Research Council, and Social Sciences and Humanities Research Council, *Memorandum of Understanding: Roles and Responsibilities in the Management of Federal Grants and Awards*, June 2002 [*Memorandum of Understanding*] at MOU-6.

89 *CIHR Act*, s. 5(d).

90 *Memorandum of Understanding* at MOU-5 and S2-2.

91 *Brown v. British Columbia (Minister of Transportation and Highways)*, [1994] 1 S.C.R. 420.

92 As the issue of causation cannot be discussed in the abstract, I cannot give a full analysis of this element. The reader should keep in mind that causation might be founded on the 'but for' test, the 'material contribution' test, or via a 'loss of chance' doctrine, depending on the circumstances.

93 [1994] 1 S.C.R. 445.

94 [1992] 1 F.C. 408 (C.A.).

95 Robert Steinbrook, 'Improving Protection for Research Subjects' (2002) 346 New Eng. J. Med. 1425 at 1427.

96 *Regulatory Impact Analysis Statement* at 1143.

Contributors

James Robert Brown is a professor of philosophy at the University of Toronto. His interests cover a variety of issues connected to the nature of science. His books have focused on topics such as thought experiments, visualization in mathematical reasoning, scientific realism, and the science-society relationship. The last topic mentioned is the subject of his most recent book, *Who Rules in Science? A Guide to the Wars*.

Lorraine E. Ferris (PhD, C.Psych, LLM) is a Professor of Public Health Sciences in the Faculty of Medicine, University of Toronto; a senior scientist, Clinical Epidemiology Unit, Sunnybrook and Women's College Health Sciences Centre and in the Institute for Clinical Evaluative Sciences (ICES); and the academic advisor, judicial affairs and policy, to the dean of medicine and vice-provost (Relations with Health Care Institutions), University of Toronto. Dr Ferris's scholarly work focuses on health services research, women's health, and medico-legal-policy issues – especially as these pertain to public protection – in areas such as standards of medical care, confidentiality, professional regulation, and research environments. She is the vice-chair of the Ethics Committee for the World Association of Medical Editors and is on the editorial board for Risk Management in Canadian Health Care. She has over eighty scholarly publications.

Paul L. Gelsinger is the father of Jesse Gelsinger, whose tragic death on 17 September 1999 led to the re-examination of policies relating to the protection of patients in gene therapy trials. Paul continues to actively support groups such as the National Organization for Rare Disorders in New Fairfield, Connecticut, and Citizens for Responsible

Care and Research (CIRCARE), an advocacy group in New York City. He is now serving a two-year term as vice-president of CIRCARE, a non-profit national organization of concerned professionals and lay persons whose common goal is to improve the safeguards for human research subjects. He is also a member of the board of directors of PHRP (Partnership for Human Research Protections), a joint venture by JCAHO (Joint Commission on Accreditation of Healthcare Organizations) and NCQA (National Committee for Quality Assurance) that accredits research institutions and IRBs.

Kathleen Cranley Glass, LLB, BCL, DCL, is director of McGill University's Biomedical Ethics Unit, associate professor in the Departments of Human Genetics and Pediatrics, and clinical ethicist at the Montreal Children's Hospital. Dr Glass holds a master's degree in political science from the University of Chicago, a doctorate in health law and ethics from the Institute of Comparative Law at McGill, and has been a visiting fellow at the Division of Medical Ethics at Harvard. She is a member of the CIHR Institute of Human Development, Child and Youth Health, the Ethics, Law and Social Issues Committee of the Canadian Longitudinal Health Initiative, and served on the Health Canada/CIHR National Placebo Working Committee. Dr Glass has published widely on issues of consent and risk with special populations – children, the elderly, psychiatric patients and research participants – as well as ethical and legal issues in clinical trials.

Sana Halwani, BSc (Hon) (Queen's), MA (Sheffield), JD (Toronto), was called to the bar of Ontario in 2005. Ms Halwani graduated from the Faculty of Law, University of Toronto, with Honours and was awarded the Dean's Key. She articled for Gilbert's LLP, a law firm in downtown Toronto with expertise in the pharmaceutical industry, and is clerking for Justice Rosalie Abella, Supreme Court of Canada, in 2005–6.

Jeffrey Kahn, PhD (Georgetown), MPH (Johns Hopkins), holds the Maas Family Endowed Chair in Bioethics and is director of the Center for Bioethics at the University of Minnesota, where he has been on the faculty since 1996. He is also professor in the Department of Medicine, Medical School; Division of Health Services Research and Policy, School of Public Health; and in the Department of Philosophy. Dr Kahn served as associate director of the White House Advisory Committee on Human Radiation Experiments (1994–5), while on the faculty of the Medical College of Wisconsin. He publishes widely in both the medical and bioethics literature, serves on numerous state and federal advisory panels, and speaks nationally and internationally on a range of bioethics topics. From 1998 through 2002 he wrote the bi-weekly bioethics column 'Ethics Matters' on CNN.com. He currently chairs the University of Minnesota Stem Cell Ethics Advisory Board.

Sheldon Krimsky is professor of Urban & Environmental Policy & Planning and adjunct professor in the Department of Public Health and Family Medicine at Tufts University. He received his bachelors and masters degrees in physics from Brooklyn College, CUNY and Purdue University respectively, and a masters and doctorate in philosophy at Boston University. Professor Krimsky's research has focused on the linkages between science/technology, ethics/values, and public policy. He is the author of eight books and has published over 150 articles and reviews. His published books include: *Genetic Alchemy: The Social History of the Recombinant DNA Controversy; Biotechnics and Society: The Rise of Industrial Genetics; Hormonal Chaos: The Scientific and Social Origins of the Environmental Endocrine Hypothesis;* and *Science in the Private Interest: Has the Lure of Profits Corrupted Biomedical Research?*

Trudo Lemmens, Lic Jur (Leuven), LLM, DCL (McGill) is associate professor in the Faculty of Law at the University of Toronto, with cross-appointments in Medical Genetics and Microbiology and Psychiatry. His teaching and research currently focus on health law and policy and bioethics, especially regulatory and ethical issues of medical research, and on legal and ethical issues raised in the area of biotechnology. He has chaired and been a member of various advisory and ethics committees and has been regularly involved in drafting reports for provincial and federal governments and governmental agencies in his areas of expertise.

Anna Mastroianni, JD, MPH, is assistant professor of law at the University of Washington. She teaches health law and bioethics in the School of Law, the Institute for Public Health Genetics, the School of Public Health and Community Medicine (Dept. of Health Services), and the School of Medicine (Dept. of Medical History and Ethics) at the University of Washington in Seattle. She has held a number of legal and governmental policy positions in Washington, DC, including associate director of the White House Advisory Committee on Human Radiation Experiments and study director of the Institute of Medicine. As a practising health care attorney, her clients included health care facilities, providers, and managers. She has been nationally recognized for her contributions to health policy, law, and bioethics by the American Association for the Advancement of Science. Her publications include four books and numerous articles concerning biomedical research and public health policy.

Paul B. Miller, BA (Mt Allison), MA (Toronto), MPhil (Cambridge), JD (Toronto), is a PhD candidate in philosophy at the University of Toronto. Mr Miller's doctoral thesis is a philosophical exploration of the law of fiduciary obligation. His research has resulted in publications in journals including the *American Journal of Bioethics*, the *Hastings Center Report*, the *Kennedy Institute of Ethics Journal*, the *Journal of Law Medicine & Ethics*, the *Pharmacogenomics Journal*, and *Nature Medicine*. Mr Miller's research is supported by a doctoral fellowship from the Social Sciences and Humanities Research Council of Canada.

C. David Naylor has recently been appointed as fifteenth President of the University of Toronto. He has been dean of the Faculty of Medicine and vice-provost (Relations with Health Care Institutions) at the University of Toronto since 1999. He previously served as founding director of Clinical Epidemiology at Sunnybrook Health Science Centre (1990–6) and founding chief executive officer of the Institute for Clinical Evaluative Sciences (1991–8). In 2003 Naylor chaired the National Advisory committee on SARS and Public Health. The committee's report catalyzed the creation of the Public Health Agency of Canada, a major federal investment in a national immunization strategy, and the appointment of Canada's first chief public health officer. Naylor has received national and international awards for scholarship and leadership in the health field, including, most recently, election to fellowship in the Royal Society of Canada.

Mary M. Thomson, BA (Hons.), MA, LLB, is one of Canada's preeminent practitioners in the areas of pharmaceutical and health law, mass tort litigation, products liability, consent law, medical negligence, and privacy issues in the health care field. She is a senior partner in the litigation department of McCarthy Tétrault LLP, based in the Toronto office, and has represented clients before the courts, commissions of inquiry, professional regulatory bodies, and other administrative tribunals. She has authored articles and papers on a variety of topics. She currently lectures on 'Ethical and Legal Issues in the Health Law Field' in the Graduate Department of Health Administration, Faculty of Medicine, University of Toronto, and throughout her career has taught advanced Trial Advocacy at the University of Toronto and the Intensive Trial Advocacy Workshop at Osgoode Hall Law School.

Duff R. Waring, BA, MA, LLB, PhD, is an assistant professor of Philosophy at York University, Toronto, where he teaches in the areas of ethical theory, bioethics, social philosophy, and critical reasoning. His current research interests involve the philosophy of psychiatry. He has published in the *Journal of Law and Social Policy*, *Canada's Mental Health*, the *Journal of Mind and Behavior*, *Bioethics*, *Theoretical Medicine and Bioethics*, and the *American Journal of Bioethics*. He articled with the Policy Development Division of the Ministry of the Attorney General, and was admitted to the Law Society of Upper Canada in 1987. He then worked for nine years at the Psychiatric Patient Advocate Office of Ontario. In 1993, he received the David J. Vail National Advocacy Award from the National Health Association of Minnesota and the U.S. National Association for Rights Protection and Advocacy. In 2002, he was awarded the Governor General's Academic Medal for his doctoral work at York University. His book, *Medical Benefit and the Human Lottery: An Egalitarian Approach to Patient Selection*, was published in 2005.

Index